Marijuana
Medical
Handbook

Practical Guide to the Therapeutic Uses of Marijuana

Dale Gieringer, Ph.D., Ed Rosenthal,
Gregory T. Carter, M.D.

Published by Quick American, Oakland, California
Editorial Assistants:
        Emily Peacock
        Anna Foster
Cover and Interior Design: Blue Hera Design
Copyright © 2008 by Quick Trading Co.

Publisher's Cataloging-in-Publication
(Provided by Quality Books, Inc.)

        Gieringer, Dale H.
        Marijuana medical handbook : practical guide to the
        therapeutic uses of marijuana / Dale Gieringer, Ed
        Rosenthal, Gregory T. Carter. -- Rev. ed.
        p. cm.
        Rev. ed. of: Marijuana medical handbook / Ed
        Rosenthal, Tod Mikuriya, Dale Gieringer.
        Includes bibliographical references and index.
        ISBN-13: 978-0-932551-86-3
        ISBN-10: 0-932551-86-6
        Printed in Canada
        1. Marijuana--Therapeutic use--Handbooks, manuals,
        etc. 2. Cannabis--Therapeutic use--Handbooks, manuals,
        etc. I. Rosenthal, Ed. II. Carter, Gregory T. III. Rosenthal,
        Ed. Marijuana medical handbook. IV. Title.

        RM666.C266R68 2008   615'.7827
                        QBI08-600186

Dedication

Dedicated to Tod Mikuriya, M.D. (1933–2007),
pioneering medical cannabis practitioner and coauthor of
the first edition of *Marijuana Medical Handbook*, whose
clinical observations and data on over 9000 patients
provided an invaluable basis for this book.

Acknowledgements

*We would like to acknowledge Paul Armentano,
Dr. Franjo Grotenhermen, Dr. Ethan Russo,
Dr. Robert Melamede, Dr. Thomas O'Connell,
Arno Hazekamp, Valerie Corral, Rick Pfrommer and
Harborside Health Center for their assistance.*

ONGOING DEVELOPMENTS: *Research on marijuana's medical use advances
constantly. Current developments along with legal and policy changes are
posted at www.norml.org*

Table of Contents

Forward to the Second Edition

The ten years since the first edition of this book appeared have witnessed exciting advances in medical marijuana. At that time, the voters of California had just approved the first state law legalizing medical marijuana, the Compassionate Use Act of 1996 (Proposition 215)[1]. Since then, 11 more states have approved medical marijuana laws, as have Canada, Austria and the Netherlands, and a growing tide of other states and nations are moving toward similar legislation.

Ten years of research have validated many findings that we tentatively outlined in the first edition of this book, at that time based on anecdotal reports. New clinical studies have found that marijuana and its ingredients are effective in treating symptoms of HIV/AIDS, multiple sclerosis, chronic and acute pain, and Tourette's syndrome. Other studies have pointed toward a host of new applications, including gastro-intestinal disorders, rheumatoid arthritis, fibromyalgia, ALS, hepatitis C, perhaps even diabetes, Alzheimer's and cancer. New biochemical research has improved our understanding of cannabinoids, illuminating their anti-inflammatory, analgesic, immuno-modulatory, neuro-protective, and anti-tumorogenic properties.

Meanwhile, the practice of cannabis medicine has vastly expanded. Over 300,000 Americans are now using marijuana under state medical marijuana laws. This is actually just the tip of the iceberg, as surveys indicate the potential U.S. patient population could be over three million. Thousands of physicians are now recommending marijuana under state medical marijuana laws. Despite the federal government's efforts to suppress them, hundreds of cannabis dispensaries and patients' coops have sprung up to supply medicine to patients in California and elsewhere.

The past decade has also seen important advances in the development of new methods for administering cannabis. Vaporizers that effectively eliminate the toxins from marijuana smoke have been developed. In the

---

1 Arizonans also approved a medical marijuana law, Prop. 200, in 1996, but it had no effect due to improper wording.

UK, GW Pharmaceuticals has developed a pharmaceutical spray made from natural cannabis extract that is now legally approved in Canada and also available to certain patients in 22 other countries.

Unfortunately, one thing has not changed, and that is the U.S. government's obstinate opposition to medical marijuana. Despite the overwhelming evidence of its medical efficacy, marijuana remains firmly classified as an illegal, Schedule I drug – that is, one with no (government-acknowledged) medical value. In 1999, the National Institute of Medicine issued a report on medical marijuana finding that it had unique benefits and urging further research, but its conclusions were ignored. The Supreme Court has twice rejected legal challenges to the federal laws against medical marijuana. The U.S. Justice Department and Drug Enforcement Administration (DEA) have launched scores of raids, arrests, and prosecutions against medical marijuana providers and growers in California and elsewhere. The DEA has even gone so far as to obstruct research into medical marijuana, blocking approval of new production facilities that would allow marijuana to be developed as an FDA-approved drug. As a result, marijuana remains no closer to FDA approval today than it was ten years ago.

It would be foolhardy to predict when the federal government will come to its senses and legalize medical marijuana, though logic would dictate that it should be legalized soon. In the meantime, there is no valid reason for Americans or anyone else to be denied the benefits of this valuable medicine. Ten years from now, countless more will be using medical marijuana than today.

This book is written for the sake of those interested in better understanding and exploring this natural, home-grown medicine.

Chapter 1
How Safe is Marijuana?

Marijuana is a remarkably safe drug. Although its primary active ingredients (THC and other cannabinoids) produce psychoactive effects at doses of a couple of milligrams, they do not have lethal effects. Unlike other psychoactive drugs, including alcohol, aspirin, opiates, nicotine, and caffeine, cannabis is not known to cause fatal overdoses. The DEA's [Drug Enforcement Administration] own administrative judge Francis Young, in his 1988 decision recommending legalization of medical marijuana, wrote, "Marijuana, in its natural form, is one of the safest therapeutically active substances known to mankind." From animal experiments, it has been estimated that a lethal dose of cannabis would be 20,000 to 40,000 times a normal dose: approximately 40 to 80 pounds of marijuana! No deaths from cannabis overdose have ever been recorded.

Marijuana's safety may be explained by how it acts in the body. In recent years, scientists have discovered that marijuana's active ingredients, the cannabinoids, work on a signaling system in our bodies known as the endogenous cannabinoid, or endocannabinoid system. Receptor cells for this system are concentrated in many parts of the brain and body, but are relatively lacking in the brainstem, which controls vital functions such as breathing and heartbeat. Therefore, even strong doses do not endanger life.

This is not to say that marijuana cannot have adverse effects. Like all drugs, marijuana can cause harm if taken in excess or abused. In addition, certain people simply respond poorly to marijuana,

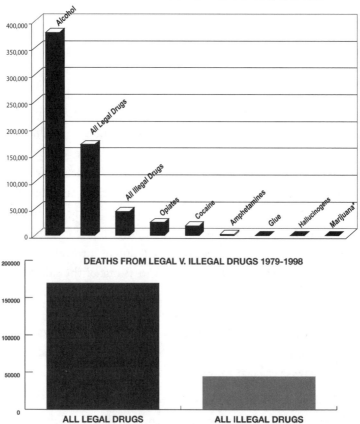

Source: *Centers for Disease Control, cited at http://briancbennett.com/charts/death/ rec-intox-deaths.htm*

finding it more unpleasant than beneficial. But what's important is that people have access to accurate information about marijuana. Without information, how will they know whether it will benefit them, what dose they should take, and how they can gain access to a regular supply?

History of Marijuana as Medicine

Marijuana, botanically known as cannabis, has been around for thousands of years. It has several species or varieties, most notably cannabis sativa and cannabis indica. Until 1937, marijuana was legal and was commonly prescribed medicinally in the U.S. Despite its prohibition, marijuana continues to be one of the most widely used drugs in America.

The medical and recreational uses of cannabis have been known since ancient times. In China, it appears in the Pen Ts'ao as a remedy for "gout, rheumatism, malaria, beriberi, constipation, and absentmindedness." Tradition ascribes the Pen Ts'ao to the legendary emperor Shen-Nung, said to be from the 3rd millennium BC, although modern scholarship dates it to the 1st century AD. The famous surgeon Hua T'o allegedly used cannabis to perform painless operations in the second century A.D. Eastern Indian documents in the Atharveda, dating from before the first millennium BC, also refer to the medicinal use of cannabis.

Cannabis was mentioned in medicinal texts by the ancient Assyrians, who referred to the hemp plant as "qunnabu," an apparent etymological cognate of "cannabis." Some Biblical scholars believe this is the same as the plant "kaneh bosm" (translated as "aromatic cane") in Exodus 30:23, where God directs Moses to make a holy oil composed of cinnamon, kaneh bosm and kassia [Russo[1]].

---

1 Russo E, "History of Cannabis and Its Preparations in Saga, Science, and Sobriquet," in

In the Roman world, cannabis was described in the classic medical writings of Galen and Dioscorides, who imaginatively recommended the "juice of the seed" to prevent earaches and diminishing sexual desires, and flatulence. It was also regularly prescribed as an analgesic or painkiller[2].

The oldest archeological evidence of medical use of cannabis dates from the discovery, in 1994, of an Egyptian tomb of the third century A.D. In the tomb were the remains of a young girl who had died in childbirth, accompanied by traces of hashish, or concentrated cannabis resin, which had apparently been used to ease the difficulties of labor.

An Irish physician, William B. O'Shaughnessy, brought knowledge of the medical properties of cannabis to Europe in 1839. He observed its use in India, then experimented with alcohol-based cannabis tinctures to treat rheumatism, rabies, cholera, tetanus, and convulsions. He described it as an analgesic and an "anti-convulsive remedy of the greatest value." In Victorian times, cannabis came to be popular in the treatment of painful menstruation and childbirth, asthma, migraines, neuralgia, and senile insomnia. By the late nineteenth century, however, its use began to wane as stronger and more conventional medicines became available.

Marijuana's use as a legal medicine was ended by a political misfortune. In 1937, the Marihuana Tax Act, a bill to ban marijuana, was brought before Congress. The director of the Federal Bureau of Narcotics, Harry Anslinger (who was, by the way, a former Prohibition official), led the attack on marijuana with bogus charges of madness and violence that focused on Hispanics, African Americans, and other minorities.

Chemistry and Biodiversity, 4:1614-48 (2007).

2 In fact, cannabis seeds have no known medically active ingredients, though they have been used for human nutrition and animal feed since time immemorial. Hemp seed yields nutritious edible oil that is high in linolenic acid and is also useful for cosmetic and industrial uses.

One of the most vocal groups to oppose the bill was the American Medical Association (AMA). Dr. William Woodward, the AMA's spokesperson, argued that cannabis was not dangerous and that its medicinal use would be severely curtailed by the proposed measures. The Prohibitionists prevailed through the use of a well-organized campaign of misinformation, and marijuana has been functionally illegal in the U.S. ever since.

The Marihuana Tax Act of 1937 essentially ended the medicinal use of cannabis. In 1941, it was withdrawn from the U.S. pharmaceutical market because of the burdensome requirements of the law.

Nonetheless, government sponsored panels of medical experts continued to find marijuana harmless and even potentially useful. In 1944 an expert panel of the New York Academy of Medicine organized by New York City Mayor Fiorello LaGuardia concluded that marijuana was not addictive, did not lead to abuse of other drugs, and that public hysteria about it was unfounded. Commissioner Anslinger vigorously denounced the report, and sought to destroy as many copies as possible. In 1971, President Nixon appointed the Presidential Commission on Marihuana and Drug Abuse, led by Pennsylvania Governor William Shafer. When the commission unexpectedly recommended the repeal of laws against adult use of marijuana, Nixon promptly disavowed their report. Another study by the National Academy of Sciences came to similar conclusions in 1982, and was likewise ignored by President Reagan.

The medicinal value of marijuana was rediscovered during the recreational marijuana boom of the Sixties. In the early 1970s, it was reported that some young cancer patients found that smoking a joint could relieve the gut-wrenching nausea that resulted from chemotherapy. Clinical studies at Harvard and elsewhere soon confirmed marijuana's anti-nausea properties.

Meanwhile, other patients were discovering that marijuana could help relieve glaucoma, chronic pain and muscle spasticity from spinal injuries and multiple sclerosis, and other complaints.

Interest in the medical benefits of marijuana peaked in the late 1970s, when over 35 states passed legislation to establish medical marijuana research programs. Each program was eventually smothered by federal drug regulations, which made it virtually impossible to conduct scientific medical marijuana research.

Under the terms of the 1970 Controlled Substances Act, marijuana is classified as a Schedule 1 controlled substance, meaning that it has high abuse potential and no recognized medical use. Schedule 1 drugs cannot be used without explicit permission from the DEA and the Food and Drug Administration (FDA), which involves exhaustive paperwork, long delays, and almost certain refusal.

In 1972, the National Organization for the Reform of Marijuana Laws (NORML) petitioned the government to make marijuana a Schedule 2 drug, which would allow its medical use. This action developed into a lawsuit that dragged on for 20 years and ended in defeat for NORML. In the meantime, frustrated patients were forced to seek other legal remedies.

In 1976, Robert Randall, a glaucoma patient, succeeded in persuading the federal government to supply him with marijuana under a new FDA "Compassionate Use" protocol. With the support of his physician, Randall argued that marijuana was the only drug that would prevent him from going blind and won a lawsuit against the federal government. The government grudgingly agreed to supply Randall with free marijuana from its own research farm in Mississippi. In later years, more patients managed to enroll in the Compassionate Use program, which required elaborate, time-consuming paperwork from their physicians. Pressed by a flood of over 100 new applicants who had been struck by the AIDS virus, the government closed the program to new applicants in 1991. Today, just four surviving patients still receive marijuana legally in the U.S., for conditions including glaucoma, multiple sclerosis, and rare genetic diseases.

In 1988, following extensive testimony, DEA administrative judge Francis Young ruled that marijuana's medical benefits were "clear beyond question" and that it should be reclassified as a Schedule 2 drug. Judge Young's recommendation was promptly overruled by DEA chief John Lawn, who, despite the fact that morphine and cocaine had earned a Schedule 2 classification, expressed concern that it would send the "wrong message" about marijuana's supposed harmfulness. After further legal twists and turns, a federal appeals court upheld the DEA ban in 1993. Hence, marijuana remains a Schedule 1 drug to this day.

Still, medical marijuana has attracted growing interest from health professionals. Although the AMA switched its position on marijuana after 1937, as it became more beholden to corporate interests, its California branch, the CMA, has called for research to establish guidelines for prescription use of cannabis. Other organizations have been bolder in advocating outright legalization of medical marijuana, including:

The American Public Health Association
The American College of Physicians
The American Nurses' Association
The American Psychiatric Association
The American Academy of Family Physicians
The AIDS Life Lobby
The Physicians' Association for AIDS Care
The New England Journal of Medicine
Consumer Reports Magazine

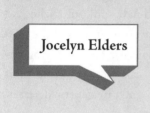

Jocelyn Elders

"It is simply wrong for the sick and suffering to be casualties in the war on drugs. Let's get rid of the myths and institute sound public-health policy."

In 1996, California voters approved an initiative that recognized the value of medical marijuana to the sick. The California Compassionate Use Act (Proposition 215) exempted patients from prosecution for possessing or cultivating marijuana for medical use if they had a physician's recommendation.

The federal government, led by Drug Czar Barry McCaffrey, attacked the initiative as contrary to federal law. The government threatened to have physicians arrested for recommending marijuana, but was blocked by a federal court decision, *Conant v. Walters*, which held that physicians were protected under the First Amendment in recommending marijuana. The government proceeded to attack medical marijuana by targeting growers, co-ops, and dispensaries providing medicine to patients, with raids that ensnared one coauthor of this book, Ed Rosenthal.

Meanwhile, in 1997, Drug Czar McCaffrey commissioned the national Institute of Medicine (IOM) to review the scientific evidence on the health benefits and risks of marijuana and drugs derived from it, known as cannabinoids. In 1999, the IOM reported that cannabinoids had "potential therapeutic value," especially for nausea reduction, appetite stimulation, anxiety reduction and pain relief. The report cautioned against use of smoked marijuana on account of the respiratory hazards of smoking, but acknowledged that it remained the only good alternative for certain patients with chronic conditions.

On Marijuana Legalization

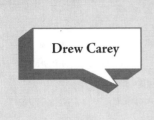
Drew Carey

"I think it's clear by now that the federal government needs to reclassify marijuana. People who need it should be able to get it safely and easily."

The report recommended further research and clinical trials including the development of non-smoked delivery systems. The federal government ignored the report and continued to oppose medical marijuana.

Despite federal opposition, support for medical marijuana grew steadily following the passage of Prop. 215. Other states passed medical marijuana laws of their own: Oregon, Washington, Alaska, Nevada, Colorado, Maine, Montana, Hawaii, Vermont, Rhode Island and New Mexico. Canada's highest court struck down the country's marijuana laws and ordered the government to institute legal access for medical users.

To this day, the U.S. government continues to insist that all use of marijuana is illegal under the federal Controlled Substances Act (CSA). In 2005, the US Supreme Court upheld this position in its ruling *Gonzalez v. Raich*. The court rejected a challenge by two California patients, Angel Raich and Diane Monson, who argued that the government's powers to regulate interstate commerce did not extend to their personal use and cultivation of medical marijuana under Prop. 215. While the court upheld the federal ban on medical marijuana, it did not question the validity of the state laws. Therefore patients are still protected from prosecution under state, though not federal, law in the 12 states with medical marijuana laws.

In practice, the DEA and Justice Department officials have insisted they have no interest in pursuing individual patients, but only

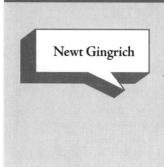

On Marijuana Legalization

Newt Gingrich

"We believe licensed physicians are competent to employ marijuana, and patients have a right to obtain marijuana legally, under medical supervision, from a regulated source. Federal policies do not reflect a factual or balanced assessment of marijuana's use as a medicant."

large-scale traffickers. As a result, most patients who possess and grow for their own individual use have little to fear so long as they are discreet and comply with local medical marijuana laws.

Since the passage of Prop. 215, public use and acceptance of medical marijuana have grown dramatically. As of this writing, some 300,000 Americans are using marijuana legally. A 2002 Time magazine poll reported that 80% of Americans support legalizing medical marijuana. It is probably only a matter of time before federal law is reformed to restore the right of U.S. citizens to use medical marijuana.

Chapter 2
What Marijuana Does

Marijuana is primarily a psychoactive, or consciousness-altering, drug. Therapeutically, its effects are wide-ranging and substantial, while physical side effects are modest and often negligible.

Marijuana acts primarily through a family of chemicals known as cannabinoids, the most prominent and psychoactive of which is delta-9-tetrahydrocannabinol or THC. THC's primary site of action is the brain, particularly the higher brain centers that affect consciousness. Cannabinoid receptors are concentrated especially in the hippocampus, which affects the higher functions of memory, feelings, and action. By acting on these higher brain systems, marijuana produces some of its most striking medicinal benefits, affecting perception of pain, mood, hunger, and muscle control. Marijuana may also produce more subtle medical effects through direct action on bodily tissues, such as immune system cells.

Marijuana users commonly report pleasurable sensations; after all, that's why people use it recreationally. There are also people who find it makes them uncomfortable. In practice, its effects on different people and in different circumstances vary, depending on individual temperament, physiology, mood, and the famous "set and setting" defined by Dr. Timothy Leary: the initial mind set of the user and the surroundings in which the user gets high.

Here are some of the more commonly reported impressions of "being high" on cannabis:

+ Heightened attentiveness to sensory stimuli, especially touch, taste, and sound; heightened interest in food and in music.

+ Free flow of ideas in rapid, loose, dreamlike succession.

+ Mild hallucinations with a "double consciousness" that some resemblances or connections are perceived, not real.

+ Disruption of concentration and short-term memory.

+ A sense of floating, light-headedness, or dizziness, and/or a sense of heaviness in the trunk and limbs.

+ Hyperactivity, restlessness, hilarity, and talkativeness for the first hour or two, followed by sleepiness and/or torpor after two to six hours.

+ Subjective "time expansion," a tendency to overestimate the amount of time that has passed.

+ Impaired executive decision-making and coordination, especially when performing complex tasks; confusion; difficulty expressing thoughts in words; slurred speech.

Chemical Composition of Marijuana

The peculiar medicinal and psychoactive effects of marijuana are primarily caused by the cannabinoids, which are a unique constituent of the marijuana plant. So far 86 cannabinoids have been identified in nature. Others have been chemically synthesized.

The main psychoactive ingredient in marijuana is delta-9-tetrahydrocannabinol, or THC (sometimes confusingly referred to as delta-1-THC under a different naming system). However, other cannabinoids also have medicinal and/or psychoactive properties.

Cannabidiol (CBD), cannabinol (CBN), cannabavarin (THCV), cannabigerol (CBG), cannabichromene (CBC), delta-8-THC, cannabicyclol (CBL), cannabitriol (CBT), and cannabielsoin are among the various natural cannabinoids. Most are known to have psychoactive and/or pharmacological effects, as do many other synthetic cannabinoid analogs.

Because delta-9-THC is the major psychoactive ingredient in marijuana, it is regularly used to measure the herb's potency. Typical concentrations of THC are less than 0.5% for inactive hemp, 2% to 3% for marijuana leaf, and 4% to 7% for higher-grade marijuana. The highest concentrations in the plant occur in seedless marijuana buds, known as sinsemilla, which can contain 10% to 20% or more. Even higher concentrations can be produced in extracts, tonics, and hashish (concentrated cannabis resin).

Therapeutic oral doses range from 2.5 to 20 milligrams of THC. A typical joint (1 gram of 2.5% leaf or 0.5 gram of 5% better grade) contains 25 milligrams of THC. However, over half of this amount is commonly destroyed in combustion or lost in side stream smoke. Only 15%–50% of the THC in a marijuana joint actually reaches the bloodstream, leaving the actual inhaled dose closer to 3–12 milligrams [Brenneisen[1]].

THC does not actually occur in its active form in the cannabis

---

1 Brenneisen, R. "Pharmacokinetics," in Grotenhermen and Russo, Cannabis and Cannabinoids, p. 67.

plant. Rather, it occurs in the form of an acid known as tetrahydrocannabinolic acid or THC acid (THCA). When marijuana is burned in a cigarette or heated in cooking, the THCA is quickly converted to THC in a heat-driven reaction known as decarboxylation. Compared to THC, little is known about THCA. While it is not psychoactive, it has been recently discovered to have immuno-modulatory properties, like other cannabinoids [Verhoeckx[2]].

If you eat marijuana raw, you will not feel strong psychoactive effects because the THCA will not have been converted to THC. However, as marijuana ages, some of the THCA will become decarboxylated. The marijuana resin in hashish often contains high levels of active THC.

The next most common cannabinoid is CBD. CBD is the leading cannabinoid in hemp varieties of cannabis. Unlike THC, CBD lacks noticeable psychoactive effects and does not strongly interact with the body's cannabinoid receptors. Nevertheless, there is growing evidence that CBD has valuable medical properties. CBD appears to work synergistically with THC, bolstering its medical effects while moderating its psychoactivity. CBD is thought to have anti-psychotic effects, dampening anxiety and panic reactions to THC. It is also thought to improve wakefulness and to enhance THC's activity against pain and spasticity. In mice, pretreatment with CBD increased brain levels of THC nearly 3-fold, and there is strong evidence that cannabinoids can increase the action of other drugs. Thus it seems that the cannabinoids work "in concert."

Taken by itself, CBD has anti-inflammatory, anti-anxiety, anti-epileptic, sedative and neuro-protective actions. It is also a potent

---

2 Verhoeckx K, et al, "Unheated Cannabis sativa extracts and its major compound THC-acid have potential immuno-modulating properties not mediated by CB1 and CB2 receptor coupled pathways," International Immunopharmacology 6 (2006) 656 – 665.

anti-oxidant, protecting against chemical damage due to oxidation. Recent laboratory and animal studies have suggested that CBD could protect against the development of diabetes, certain kinds of cancer, rheumatoid arthritis; brain and nerve damage due to stroke, alcoholism and Huntington's disease, and even prion infections such as "mad cow" disease. There is evidence that the dosage response to CBD is biphasic, meaning that its efficacy diminishes if the dose is too high or too low.

CBD is an essential ingredient in Sativex, the cannabis spray being developed by GW Pharmaceuticals in the UK. Sativex, which contains equal parts CBD and THC, has been approved for treatment of MS in Canada. GW is planning further research on the use of CBD in arthritis, inflammatory bowel diseases, psychotic disorders, and epilepsy.

CBD is produced alongside THC acid (THCA), the precursor of THC. In the marijuana plant, a cannabinoid called cannabigerolic acid is the precursor to both CBD and THCA. Each is produced by a different enzyme in the plant acting on cannabigerolic acid.

Since CBD and THCA are both produced from the same precursor it is difficult to produce plants that carry high levels of both of these cannabinoids. In hemp plants, the enzyme that produces THCA is inactive or lacking, leaving the plant high in CBD. Unfortunately, most domestically sold marijuana has very low levels of CBD, rarely as high as 1%. This is because commercial marijuana has been selectively bred to remove the CBD enzyme and produce plants high in THC. Hopefully, growers will develop marijuana with higher levels of CBD in coming years.

The third most common cannabinoid is CBN, which is a by product of chemical breakdown of THC. CBN has at most feeble effects psychoactively and medically. It is most commonly found in degraded, poorly preserved marijuana.

In addition to cannabinoids, marijuana contains over one hundred terpenoids, aromatic chemicals also found in pine trees, citrus, and other odoriferous plants. Terpenoids are responsible for the distinctive aroma and flavor of marijuana. Many investigators believe terpenoids also contribute significant medicinal effects. Compared to the cannabinoids, relatively little is known about the terpenoids in cannabis. We shall have more to say about them in Chapter 5 (Growing Medical Marijuana) and Chapter 9 (Choosing a Variety).

Cannabis also contains over 20 flavonoids, a family of chemicals common to plants. Some of these flavonoids, known as cannflavins, are unique to cannabis. Flavonoids are thought to have anti-inflammatory and anti-oxidant properties and may help protect against cancer and other diseases.

Experienced users have reported that different types of marijuana produce different highs and have different medical effects. The different proportions of cannabinoids, terpenoids, and flavonoids in different varieties - or even different plant samples—create these varied effects.

First-Time Use

The first use of marijuana is a special occasion. For reasons that aren't well understood, many people don't feel anything the first time they use it. They respond only the second or third time, as if it were necessary somehow to "prime" them for the experience. Some new users may actually act "stoned," but not notice it. The first-time threshold can usually be overcome by simply raising the dose. However, this greatly raises the risk of an unpleasant reaction. First-time users should proceed cautiously; they should be prepared to be incapacitated for a couple of hours.

Tolerance

Heavy marijuana users tend to develop a tolerance, or decreased sensitivity, to the effects of marijuana. Pleasant sensations such as euphoria tend to fade with heavy, regular use. On the other hand, the same may be true of undesired effects, such as an increased heart rate (tachycardia).

Less frequently, patients may develop a tolerance to the medical benefits of marijuana. Sometimes this problem can be remedied by switching to a different variety or dosage method for a while.

Furthermore, one person may be much more sensitive than another to the various components in marijuana. The bulk of research has examined reactions to THC, but not other ingredients in marijuana such as cannabinoids, terpenoids and flavonoids. Reactions to these components may vary among users, making dosing highly individualistic.

Drug Interactions

Marijuana rarely increases the toxic effects of other medicines. In this respect, it differs even from such common drugs as alcohol, which is extremely dangerous in combination with depressants, or aspirin, which is dangerous in combination with blood-thinning drugs such as Coumarin. This is yet one more example of marijuana's remarkable safety.

Certain drugs may interact with marijuana to stimulate tachycardia. These include the antidepressant nortriptyline and possibly the popular stimulant ephedrine (an ingredient in so-called "herbal ecstasy" preparations), which is also used as an anti-asthmatic medication. On the other hand, THC-induced tachycardia may be inhibited by beta-blockers such as propranolol.

Addiction

Marijuana is not physically addictive. Smokers may use it many times daily for many years, then give it up with no difficulty. When a former user is asked how he or she quit, a typical reply is "I just didn't use it any more." However, psychological addiction is possible.

When experts compare marijuana with alcohol, nicotine, cocaine, opiates, caffeine, and other psychoactive drugs, they rank it at or near the bottom of the list in terms of dependence, reinforcement, and withdrawal potential. Still, like every human pleasure, the use of marijuana can be strongly habit-forming for a certain minority.

About 10% of recreational users have trouble controlling their use. They are mostly addiction-prone people who have difficulty with other drugs as well. Persons who use marijuana to excess, to the point that they feel their use is out of control or that it interferes with their lives, may be defined as marijuana abusers. Some drug treatment programs deal with marijuana abusers, but they make up a small proportion of their clientele. Most patients in marijuana treatment programs are offenders who have been caught by the law or their schools and sentenced to treatment as an alternative to criminal punishment. A group known as Marijuana Anonymous offers help to those seeking to recover from marijuana abuse (www.marijuana-anonymous.org).

A minority of long-term, extremely heavy (several doses daily) recreational users experience subtle withdrawal symptoms when they give up marijuana. These include mild anxiety, depression, nightmares, difficulty sleeping, vivid dreams, irritability, tremors, perspiration, nausea, muscle convulsions, and restlessness. These symptoms, though mild, may persist for a few days, but are only noticeable in the heaviest users, and even then they present no real obstacle to anyone trying to quit.

Impaired Driving

What about people who drive and use marijuana? Aren't they at risk? In fact, cannabis can impair driving performance by interfering with attentiveness, short-term memory, and reaction time, particularly at heavier doses. However, its risks are notably less than those of drunken driving.

Here's what the U.S. National Highway Transportation Safety Administration (NHTSA) reported in a study, "Marijuana and Actual Driving Performance," conducted in the Netherlands [Hindrik and O'Hanion][3]. The study looked at drivers using various dosages of marijuana, on freeways and under urban driving conditions. It concluded that intoxication in drivers is "in no way unusual compared to many medicinal drugs." It found that marijuana does have some effect on driving ability, but is "not profoundly impairing." It explained this by the fact that, unlike alcohol, which encourages risky driving, marijuana appears to produce greater caution, apparently because its users are more aware of their state and better able to compensate for it.

Physical Effects

Although marijuana is very safe, this is not to say that it cannot have adverse effects. Like all drugs, marijuana can be harmful if taken in excess or abused.

The effects of marijuana are experienced almost immediately after inhaling or smoking. If ingested orally, they're delayed an

3 Hindrik WJR and O'Hanion J, "Marijuana and actual driving performance," published as Department of Transportation Report #DOT HS 808-078, 1996.

hour or more. If smoked, the effects are most pronounced for the first hour or two, declining gradually over the next three or four hours. They normally disappear after a good night's sleep. Unlike alcohol, opiates, cocaine, amphetamine, and many other drugs, pot doesn't produce unpleasant "hangover" or rebound effects–the high just fades away. A few supersensitive people may feel slightly sedated for a day or so after use.

Chronic users–those who smoke marijuana every day–may experience more prolonged, though low-level, effects, lasting days or even weeks after stopping. The reasons for this "cannabis haze" are uncertain.

One possible explanation is a buildup of residual cannabinoids in the system. THC is a highly fat-soluble drug that is absorbed by fat tissues throughout the body. Most of the cannabinoids inhaled from a joint end up somewhere other than the brain. They are then slowly transferred back into the bloodstream over a period of many days. For occasional users, the blood concentration of residual THC is minuscule. However, chronic heavy use raises the level of residual THC to levels that can be detected for 48 hours or more in the blood, while non-psychoactive breakdown metabolites of THC can be detected for days or weeks in the urine.

THC has few noticeable physical effects on the body. The following symptoms are commonly reported:

- Dryness of the throat, resulting in thirst.

- Redness of the eyes' outer coating, or conjunctiva, due to dilation of the small blood vessels there.

- Speeding of the heartbeat, or tachycardia.

- Reduction of pressure inside the eye, a benefit for glaucoma patients.

- Dilation of the upper bronchial passages of the lungs.

In addition, marijuana smoke has irritating, noxious effects on the lungs and respiratory system, just like tobacco. These are not due to cannabinoids, but to toxic by-products of burning. Fortunately, they can be eliminated by alternative ingestion methods, such as inhaling from smokeless vaporizers or by taking marijuana orally instead of inhaling it.

Marijuana in the Body

At the beginning of the 1990s, scientists learned that cannabinoids resemble a chemical that occurs naturally in the brain, and that marijuana's effects are caused by biological mechanisms affected by this natural chemical. Dr. William Devane discovered this chemical, known as "anandamide," in 1992. Anandamide (from the Sanskrit word for "bliss") was named by Devane's colleague Dr. Raphael Mechoulam, who also discovered the chemical structure of THC.

The brain and nervous system contain many different systems of biological mechanisms, called receptor systems. Receptors are sites that react to specific chemicals and produce specific reactions. The chemicals are called neurotransmitters, and the cascade of chain reactions throughout the networks of these systems is the process by which areas of the brain communicate with each other; this is how the brain works. Most drugs produce their effects by interfering with or activating the processes of specific systems. Barbiturates, for example, have a nonspecific effect on chloride ion channels; this increases the activity of a neurotransmitter called GABA; an increase in GABA activity has a sedative effect. Benzodiazepines, such as Valium®, have a specific effect on receptor sites that increase GABA activity.

Before the discovery of a cannabinoid receptor system in the ear-

21

ly 1990s, some scientists speculated that marijuana produced its effects through nonspecific action, like barbiturates. Nonspecific effects are generally broader and more dangerous than the effects produced by receptor site activation.

In fact, marijuana's effects are produced by a cannabinoid receptor system consisting of at least two cannabinoid receptor types: CB1 and CB2. CB1 receptors are located primarily in the brain, especially the hippocampus and cerebral cortex, which control memory and cognition. CB2 receptors occur primarily in the extremities (arms and legs) and in immune tissues, for example the spleen and white blood cells. Because they are concentrated in body tissues outside of the brain, they are referred to as "peripheral" receptors. The psychoactive effects of marijuana are due to its action on CB1 receptors. The CB2 receptors may be involved in other, more purely "medical" effects, such as anti-inflammatory action.

The biological actions associated with cannabinoid receptors include marijuana's effects on memory and cognition, on locomotor function, on pain, on endocrine actions, and on other biological changes, including a decrease in body temperature, changes in the heart rate, suppression of nausea and vomiting, and decrease in intraocular pressure. Scientists know to some degree how the CB1 receptors function, but have an incomplete understanding of how cannabinoceptive neurons interact with other neural systems. CB2 was discovered somewhat later than CB1, and understanding of CB2 is less complete.

Of course the cannabinoid receptor system did not evolve to respond to marijuana. As soon as the CB1 and CB2 receptors were discovered scientists knew that there must also be natural cannabinoids in the body that interact with these receptors. The body's internal cannabinoid-related neurotransmitters are referred to as endocannabinoids.

The principal endocannabinoid is called anandamide (after the Sanskrit word for bliss). Anandamide breaks down more rapidly than THC and seems to interact less strongly with the CB1 receptor. Anandamide and its receptors are found in the brains of all mammals and many other animals, and are thought to have evolved over hundreds of millions of years. A second endocannabinoid known as 2-AG (for 2-arachidonylglycerol) was discovered after anandamide, and researchers suspect there may be others.

Recent studies indicate that the endogenous cannabinoids transmit signals retrogradely or backwards. Where nerve signals are normally transmitted forward from synapses to neurons, cannabinoids send signals in the opposite direction, from the neurons back through the synapse.

Researchers are only beginning to understand the function of the endocannabinoid system. Animal studies indicate that it plays a role in regulating immunity, inflammation, neurotoxicity and trauma, blood pressure, body temperature, appetite, gastrointestinal function, analgesia, glaucoma, epilepsy, depression and stress, and even bone formation. Dr. Robert Melamede has described the function of the endocannabinoid system as "homeostatic," meaning that it tends to restore balance. Endocannabinoids tend to fine-tune biological responses upwards or downwards as needed within the range necessary to maintain healthy function. This is a good metaphor for the therapeutic effects of marijuana.

We noted earlier that heavy use of marijuana over a long period can produce a tolerance for the drug in some patients. Tolerance for marijuana develops from continued exposure to large amounts of cannabinoids; in response, the brain decreases the number of receptor sites available to bind cannabinoids. When the heavy exposure ends, the receptor sites increase back to a natural level.

Overdose and Treatment

There have been no reports of fatal cannabis overdose in humans. The safety reflects the paucity of receptors in the medullary nuclei, the part of the brain that controls respiratory and cardiovascular functions.

Heavy doses are nonetheless apt to produce unpleasant reactions. In rare cases, even moderate doses may result in acute panic reactions, characterized by anxiety, paranoia, self-consciousness, loss of self-control, wild racing thoughts, and disorientation. Fortunately, such reactions usually subside within a couple of hours. No medical treatment is necessary. Sufferers should be reassured that their discomfort will be brief. Often, pleasant and unpleasant feelings occur in alternating waves, as thoughts ebb and flow.

Panic reactions are most likely to occur in novice users with excessive doses and in unpleasant surroundings. First-time users should take care to start with small amounts and to allow themselves ample comfort and time to experience the drug.

Occasionally, marijuana can produce unpleasant physical symptoms, including headaches, dizziness, nausea, and vomiting, which may be secondary to mental anxiety and are most common at heavy doses. A few individuals experience such symptoms regularly, like an allergic reaction.

Most frequently, though, adverse physical reactions result from an overdose. Though never fatal, heavy overdoses are unpleasant and can be temporarily debilitating. Symptoms include anxiety, panic, excitement, hallucinations, and a racing heartbeat, proceeding to immobility, torpor, and unconsciousness. Fortunately, the effects are temporary and wear off after a few hours of sleep. No antidote is needed.

Overdoses occur less frequently with inhaled marijuana than

with oral ingestion, because smokers can sense immediately when they have had enough or when the drug content is too high. At most, smokers may step "one toke over the line" before finding they are too high and stopping. Oral doses are much harder to gauge. It's easy to take a multiple dose of brownies and not know what's hit you until an hour or two later.

Cannabis poisonings were more common around the turn of the last century, when medicinal preparations were dispensed in potent tonics containing hundreds of doses per fluid ounce.

The Paradoxical Effects of Marijuana

Marijuana has a "paradoxical" ability to produce precisely opposite reactions in different circumstances. Though it typically eases nausea, spasticity, pain, and insomnia, it can also aggravate them in exceptional situations or for exceptional subjects. Again, marijuana can cause euphoria, pleasure, or relaxation at one time and suffering, depression, or anxiety at another. The paradoxical nature of cannabis results from the fact that its effects are filtered through the highest centers of human consciousness. Thus the French poet Baudelaire called hashish "the mirror that magnifies," emphasizing the importance of personality as well as set and setting.

Marijuana appeals differently to different people. People who like it often use it to heighten their senses. They may smoke before eating, listening to music, watching plays or movies, or taking a walk or hike, or while spending time with others or just thinking. Many users report subjective feelings of creativity and inspiration, although these don't always stand up to later, sober analysis. Many devotees report feelings of euphoria, exhilaration, good will, empathy, and religious awe. They say marijuana helps them think about serious matters, to become introspective and spiritual, to get to the essence of things.

People who don't like marijuana complain of anxiety, self-consciousness, paranoia, social withdrawal, irritability, dysphoria, and loss of self-control. They may also find that it interferes with their ability to work, concentrate, and function.

Set and Setting

Marijuana's effects are especially responsive to variations in individual set and setting. Set is defined as what the user brings to the drug: his or her own medical situation, psychology, physiology, state of mind, and so on. Hence some patients are naturally more attuned to the therapeutic benefits of marijuana than others. Setting is the external situation in which the user takes the drug: the physical, sensory, and social environment. People who would normally find marijuana rewarding will often react unfavorably in the wrong circumstances, if they are pressed by obligations, discomfited by unpleasant company, or placed in disagreeable surroundings.

Cannabis Substitutes

While marijuana remains an illegal Schedule 1 drug, pharmaceutical companies have sought to develop legal cannabinoid substitutes. These include:

+ Marinol® (whose generic name is dronabinol), which consists of synthetically manufactured THC.

+ Sativex® (from the U.K.), a natural cannabis extract that is presently under development, and legally available in Canada.

What to Do if You Over-do

It's effectively impossible to give yourself a fatal overdose of cannabis. Still, you can get too high for comfort, especially if you eat it. If you eat a dose of pot too fast, then decide you need another before the effects of the first have fully hit you, you can end up "overstoned." Likewise if you misjudge the potency of the pot you're using.

Over-indulging in marijuana tends to heighten the side-effects of the drug. These include:

+ Rapid heartbeat

+ Feeling anxious, panicky, or paranoid

+ Dry mouth

+ Nausea and dizziness

The only cure for too much cannabis is time for your body to clear it out. This might take a few hours: a good night's sleep will put you right. However there are some things you can do to make it easier on you until it passes.

+ Remember that you're in no danger. It's easy to give in to the panic signals, but the more you worry the worse it will get. Keep telling yourself that it will pass, and it will.

+ Talk to someone. The best person to talk you through a bad high is a friend who has some experience with marijuana. Talking about how you're feeling can help you set the negative stuff apart from yourself, and an experienced friend can reinforce your knowledge that you'll be fine before long.

+ Avoid alcohol, caffeine, or other drugs. They won't make you feel any better, and they might make things a lot worse.

+ Get a cold drink. You aren't really dehydrated, but your mouth may feel like a mile of dry sand. Something cold and wet will help with that.

+ Take your mind off it as much as you can. Some sort of

mindless entertainment such as watching cartoons is a good bet.

+ If you find yourself in a place with a lot of noise and activit, try to find a quiet corner—but resist the urge to leave and go someplace else.

+ DO NOT DRIVE or operate machinery. Pot is less impairing than alcohol, but you can have an accident even on your best day. Have an accident while you're high and your problems will go on long after you come down.

+ If you can sleep, do so. Sleep is the best thing for you at this point, so try to make yourself comfortable enough to fall asleep.

+ Nabilone (a synthetic cannabinoid analogue marketed in the U.S. under the name of Cesamet®).

Marinol® (Dronabinol)–Oral Synthetic THC

By far the closest substitute for marijuana is Marinol®, generically known as dronabinal, which consists of pure THC in oral capsules. The THC is chemically synthesized by an expensive, patented process, then dissolved in sesame oil and put in soft gel capsules. At present, Marinol is marketed by Solvay Pharmaceuticals in doses of 2.5, 5, and 10 milligrams. It was introduced to the market in 1986 as an anti-nauseant for cancer chemotherapy. In 1993, it was also approved for nausea and appetite loss arising from AIDS wasting syndrome. The FDA approved both uses on the basis of controlled safety and efficacy studies.

Marinol is currently a Schedule 3 controlled substance. Originally, it was classified in Schedule 2, the most tightly controlled category. Schedule 2 prescriptions must be filed in triplicate so that the authorities can monitor them. Therefore, doctors were reluctant to prescribe Marinol. In 1999, Marinol was downgraded to Schedule 3, which does not require triplicate prescriptions. The rescheduling decision was influenced by a study from the Haight-Ashbury Free Clinic, which found that Marinol had a low abuse potential and wasn't dealt much on the illicit market. Since the rescheduling, doctors have little reason to worry about government harassment for prescribing Marinol.

The development of Marinol was promoted by federal officials in the Reagan administration in the hope of stemming medicinal demand for natural marijuana. The availability of Marinol is often cited as a reason to keep medical marijuana illegal. Its proponents argue that Marinol is preferable because it is a chemically pure pharmaceutical, produced in controlled doses, rather than a smoked herb, consisting of unknown quantities of different chemicals. In fact, Marinol has proven to be a poor and imperfect substitute for natural marijuana. Though some patients find it useful, many others report that it doesn't work as well as natural marijuana.

One limitation of Marinol is that it contains just one medically active cannabinoid, THC. It lacks all the other potentially active cannabinoids in natural marijuana, such as CBD, as well as the terpenoids and flavonoids. As we've seen, these ingredients may have unique medical benefits. As a result, pure THC may not be ideal for many patients.

Perhaps the greatest limitation of Marinol is that it comes only in oral doses. In contrast, natural marijuana can also be inhaled by smoking. Inhalation is preferable in many medical circumstances. In particular, chemotherapy patients are often so nauseated that they have trouble holding down any oral medication. The easiest way for such people to get marijuana into their systems is through inhalation.

Inhalation is also preferable when users need fast relief. Oral doses frequently take an hour or more to take effect, whereas inhaled marijuana takes effect almost at once. Patients can promptly treat a sudden attack of pain, or an oncoming seizure or muscle spasm, with smoked marijuana, but not with oral Marinol.

Another important advantage of inhalation is that it allows patients to regulate their dosage more accurately through a process known as self-titration. Once you inhale marijuana, you can sense immediately whether it has had the effect you need. If not, you can just take another puff. With oral doses, however, you have to guess the proper amount beforehand, then wait an hour or so to see whether you were right. This makes it easy to overshoot or undershoot the mark.

All of this makes nonsense of claims by opponents of marijuana that only Marinol affords scientifically controlled, well-prescribed dosages. For many purposes, such as relief of pain, discomfort, and nausea, patients are in a better position to adjust their own dose through self-titration than doctors who try to guess what oral dose is appropriate.

In fact, even though Marinol comes in well-defined doses, it is difficult to predict how much of it will be absorbed into your system. This is because the bioavailability of oral THC varies greatly according to the state of your digestive system, metabolism and other factors. The same oral dose may be insufficient on one occasion and overpowering on another. As a result, misdosage is a common problem with Marinol. In particular, patients appear to experience a high incidence of anxiety attacks due to overdose, a problem that may be aggravated by Marinol's lack of CBD.

Users report better results by dissolving a Marinol capsule under their tongues. This route, known as "sublingual" administration, allows the THC to be absorbed directly through the oral tissues into the bloodstream without having to pass through the digestive system. Sublingual administration delivers THC more rapidly (typically within 15-20 minutes) and reliably than oral ingestion. Although this route of administration seems preferable, it is discouraged by the label, which directs patients to swallow the pill.

Perversely, because Marinol is formulated with sesame oil, it is difficult to administer by inhalation. The sesame oil produces an irritating smoke when burned, and also makes Marinol impossible to vaporize.

Yet another major drawback of Marinol is its price, which is up to $1,000 per bottle of 60. Patients have been known to run through several prescriptions a month. Unless you have good insurance, this is tough medicine. Marinol is so expensive because it's chemically synthesized. As we'll see, it's possible to produce high-potency extracts of THC much more cheaply from home-grown marijuana. When cannabis was still on the pharmaceutical market in the 1920s, a one-pint bottle containing 4700 doses could be bought for as little as $4, or one tenth of a cent per dose! In our own time, when the cost of health care is a major issue, it's ironic that our government has outlawed this uniquely affordable medication.

Marinol does have some advantages. It's medically pure, so there's no risk of contamination from bacteria, fungi, pesticides, or other contaminants that can creep into black-market marijuana.

In addition, Marinol doesn't involve the respiratory hazards of smoking. Of course, neither do oral preparations of natural cannabis. However, Marinol's consistency and purity have the advantage of predictability of strength when it is taken on a continuing basis. In contrast, homemade oral preparations can vary greatly in potency from batch to batch.

The most important advantage of Marinol is its legality. Marinol can be prescribed by any physician who has a DEA license (almost all do). Like other FDA-approved drugs, it may be prescribed legally for any indication, not just those mentioned on the label. When Marinol was first approved, the DEA tried to restrict it only to use for cancer chemotherapy, but this was never enforced. Doctors are now prescribing it for a wide range of indications like marijuana. However, doctors tend to be more reluctant to prescribe it for off-label indications, especially those for which there exist no solid scientific data showing efficacy of THC. In addition, health insurance companies won't pay for prescription drugs used in off-label indications. If you want to use Marinol for anything other than nausea from cancer or weight loss from AIDS, you must pocket the hefty tab yourself.

Marinol, Marijuana, and Drug Testing

Marinol's legality has important implications for anyone who is subject to drug testing for employment, insurance, or law enforcement. So long as marijuana remains a Schedule 1 drug, you have no right to use it even medically, so you can be dismissed on the basis of a positive drug test. Since urine tests can detect marijuana metabolites in urine for one to five days after an occasional use and up to six weeks for chronic users, this poses obvious problems for medical marijuana users.

One answer to this problem is to obtain a prescription for Marinol. Because Marinol is based on THC, it is indistinguishable from marijuana on the most commonly used drug screens. Workers generally have the right to test positive for any drug legally prescribed to them. Therefore, if they have a prescription for Marinol, they can't be disqualified for a marijuana-positive test!

There are, however, limitations with this tactic. First, you will have to inform the medical review officer beforehand that you are taking Marinol. This will involve disclosing your medical condition and may give the employer an excuse not to hire you. Second, new advances in drug detection technology have made it possible to distinguish marijuana from pure THC. According to Dr. Mahmoud ElSohly, director of the government's University of Mississippi marijuana research program, it is possible to detect certain non-THC cannabinoid metabolites that are present only in natural marijuana, not in Marinol. This requires the use of expensive and sophisticated gas chromatograph mass spectrometer (GCMS) tests. You are highly unlikely to encounter such tests in the normal course of events. The standard drug screens are completely incapable of distinguishing between Marinol and marijuana. If, however, you arouse unusual suspicions, it is possible that you could be subjected to a more probing investigation. This has been done in the federal court system to prevent medical marijuana defendants from using anything but Marinol while in custody.

Sativex®: Cannabis Extract Spray

Additional new pharmaceuticals based on natural cannabis extracts are under development by a British company, GW Pharmaceuticals. One of them, Sativex®, has already been approved in Canada for treatment of multiple sclerosis, and is also available for special patients in 22 other countries. Sativex is in the early stages of testing in the U.S.

Sativex is an oral spray consisting of equal parts THC and CBD extracted from marijuana grown by GW Pharmaceuticals. Under the direction of Dr. Geoffrey Guy, an expert on herbal medicines, GW operates the most advanced marijuana growing facility in the world, a climate-controlled indoor garden at a secret location in southern England. The garden features many unique varieties with varying concentrations of different cannabinoids. By blending different plant extracts, GW Pharmaceuticals is able to experiment with many different combinations of cannabinoids.

Sativex differs from Marinol in important ways. First, it incorporates CBD and other plant ingredients as well as THC. GW says that its research showed the mixture is more effective, partly because CBD mitigated untoward psychoactive effects of pure THC. Sativex was first developed for treating symptoms of MS, but is also being tested for neuropathic pain from spinal cord injury, cancer, and diabetes. GW is also developing a higher-CBD product for rheumatoid arthritis, inflammatory bowel diseases, epilepsy and psychotic disorders, and a high-THC product for chronic pain.

Second, Sativex is not a pill, but a spray delivered under the tongue. This delivery method is not as fast as inhalation, as it still takes several minutes for the cannabinoids to be absorbed through the membranes of the mouth. However, it is faster than oral ingestion. It also delivers a far more consistent dosage, since the cannabinoids are absorbed directly into the blood from the oral membranes without having to pass through the digestive system.

Third, Sativex is cheaper to manufacture because the cannabinoids are derived from the plant rather than expensive chemical synthesis. Of course, Sativex will never be as cheap as natural marijuana, which you can grow in your own home garden!

Due to the inordinate delay of FDA and DEA drug bureaucrats, it will be several years before American consumers are free to obtain Sativex or other state-of-the-art cannabis pharmaceuticals. When they arrive, they will offer a valuable new alternative for patients in need of cannabis therapy. Still, it is unlikely that any pharmaceutical drug will ever displace natural, homegrown marijuana.

Nabilone: A non-natural cannabinoid analogue

As interest in cannabis medicine has grown, pharmaceutical companies have explored the development of new, synthetic drugs based on cannabinoids. From the standpoint of the industry, such new "analogue" drugs have the advantage of being easy to patent, unlike the cannabinoids that occur in nature. On the other hand, they also bear a higher risk of unsuspected adverse reactions because they have not been in usage very long.

Nabilone is a synthetic cannabinoid that was introduced to the market in the U.K. for treatment of nausea from chemotherapy during the 1980s. More recently, it has been tested for treatment of pain and movement disorders. In 2006, nabilone was finally introduced to the U.S. market under the trade name of Cesamet®. Like most cannabinoid analogues, nabilone lacks the distinctive psychoactive properties of THC, both adverse and beneficial, and has not gained widespread usage. Other synthetic cannabinoid analogues, such as levonatrodol and synhexyl, have been tested over the years but never reached the market. Many new synthetic cannabinoids are under investigation, some of which have proven useful for laboratory research purposes.

Rimonabant: the "Anti-Pot" Pill

Amidst the resurgent interest in cannabis medicine, drug companies have begun to explore a number of new synthetic drugs aimed at targeting the cannabinoid receptors. One of the more interesting is rimonabant, which functions as a kind of "anti-pot" drug by antagonizing or interfering with the CB1 receptor.

The French company Sanofi-Aventis developed rimonabant as a diet drug, under the trade name Accomplia®. That an anti-marijuana drug would be considered for weight loss is hardly surprising, given marijuana's reputation for stimulating appetite and causing the munchies. The problem, of course, is that it might also be expected to reverse marijuana's many other medical benefits for pain, spasticity, inflammation, glaucoma, auto-immune disease, mood disorders, etc.

Surprisingly, even though Accomplia® was a new chemical without a long safety record, regulatory authorities in Europe, Brazil, Argentina, Mexico and elsewhere quickly approved it. In contrast, marijuana, with a centuries-long record of proven safety and efficacy, remains illegal. This is a testimony to the bias of mainstream medicine in favor of synthetic pharmaceuticals.

In corporate pharmaceutical circles, Accomplia® was touted as a blockbuster drug. In clinical trials, it helped subjects lose a significant amount of weight – 14 pounds in one year and 2.4 pounds more the second year. After discontinuing the drug, however, they gained the weight back, implying that they would have to keep taking it indefinitely in order to retain the benefits.

Rimonabant's "Slenderella" story came to an end in 2007, when the U.S. FDA denied approval of the drug for very good reasons that could have been anticipated. It was noted that rimonabant was linked to suicidal thoughts, depression, anxiety and nausea – the very kind of dysphoric reactions one might expect from an "anti-pot." Rimonabant was also reported to induce symptoms of multiple sclerosis – the tip of a likely iceberg of other untoward reactions due to blocking the CB1 receptor. Newborn mice injected with rimonabant refused feeding and tended to die. Genetically altered mice lacking cannabinoid receptors suffer numerous health defects, including oversensitivity to pain, decreased activity and increased mortality. In sum, the saga of rimonabant is a poignant reminder of the dangers of blocking the body's cannabinoid system.

Chapter 3
Medicinal Uses of Marijuana

Scientific evidence for marijuana's efficacy in treating a wide range of diseases is increasing by the day. In recent years, rigorous, double-blind studies have found cannabis or natural cannabis extracts to be effective for treating nausea and appetite loss from cancer chemotherapy, pain and appetite loss due to HIV/AIDS, multiple sclerosis, and other conditions. Many other uses have been reported in less rigorous clinical studies, surveys, and anecdotal reports. Remarkably, only mild temporary adverse side effects, at worst, have been reported and no serious toxic reactions were found in any case, a record unheard of for most pharmaceutical drugs. Medical cannabis specialist Dr. Tod Mikuriya has reported over 200 separate indications or uses for medical cannabis (See Appendix, Table 1). These can be broken down into the following broad categories

+ Anti-nauseant and appetite stimulant
+ Anti-spasmodic and anti-convulsant

+ Analgesic (pain reliever)

+ Anti-inflammatory and immune system modulator

+ Anxiolytic (anxiety reliever) and anti-depressant for mood disorders

+ Harm reduction substitute for alcohol, opiates and other dangerous drugs

+ Miscellaneous applications like glaucoma and asthma

SPECIFIC USES FOR MEDICAL MARIJUANA:
Anti-nauseant and Appetite Stimulant

The most familiar and longest-established use of cannabis in modern medicine is as an anti-nauseant or antiemetic—that is, a treatment for severe nausea and vomiting. In particular, marijuana is widely used in connection with cancer chemotherapy and radiation therapy, which can cause intense nausea.

Cannabis has been known to suppress nausea and stimulate appetite since its introduction to modern medicine in the nineteenth century. Recreational users have long been familiar with the "munchies," a heightened appetite (usually for snacking) that overtakes many users shortly after smoking.

Paradoxically, at high doses, cannabis can sometimes precipitate nausea. Toxic reactions of this sort result from oral overdoses of the kind indulged in by the more adventurous hashish eaters.

The use of marijuana to treat anorexia (loss of weight and appetite) associated with radiation and chemotherapy was documented in the early 1970s. At that time, chemotherapy, like marijuana, was emerging into widespread use. Radiation and chemotherapy drugs are by nature quite toxic, producing a more profound nausea than any associated with common diseases. Following their administration, patients can suffer hours of gut-wrenching vomiting, with "dry heaves" so severe as to result in broken bones. Nausea can persist for days or even weeks, leaving patients unable to eat. The distress can be so severe that some patients choose to forgo treatment altogether rather than endure it. A number of drugs are available by prescription for control of the side effects of radiation medicine and chemotherapy, but they're not always satisfactory and can be extremely expensive.

Many patients find that a joint can relieve the misery of radiation medicine and chemotherapy better than any other medicine. The remarkable value of marijuana was discovered serendipitously by young radiation and chemotherapy patients familiar with its recreational use. Their stories came to the attention of doctors at Harvard University, among them Dr. Lester Grinspoon, whose own son Danny used it to treat himself during cancer chemotherapy. A flurry of research soon followed, in which both marijuana and oral THC were found to be effective in reducing nausea and vomiting from chemotherapy. Interest peaked in the early 1980s, when a number of states sponsored clinical research studies of medical marijuana.

In all, smoked marijuana was shown to be an effective anti-nauseant in six different state studies: New Mexico (250 patients), New York (199), California (98), Tennessee (27), Georgia (119), and Michigan (165) [Randall[1]].

In New Mexico, New York, and Tennessee, smoked marijuana proved to be effective in 90% of patients; in Georgia and Tennessee, it was effective in over 70%. In New Mexico and Tennessee, smoked marijuana also proved superior to oral THC. In Michigan, patients found smoked marijuana preferable to a conven-

---

[1] For a summary of the state studies on marijuana for cancer chemotherapy, see Robert Randall, ed., Marijuana, Medicine and the Law, Vol. 2 (Galen Press, Wash. DC) 1989, pp. 36ff.

tional prescription anti-nauseant, Torecan®. In both New York and Tennessee, marijuana was effective for patients who had not been helped by THC.

The California study, which focused largely on oral THC, produced the weakest evidence for marijuana. Still, it found marijuana to be effective in 59% of patients, about the same as oral THC (57%). However, only 17% rated marijuana "highly effective," versus 30% for oral THC. About 11% of patients dropped out of treatment because of side effects, including anxiety, confusion, dizziness, depression, perceptual distortion, and so on. (Remarkably, "euphoria" was mentioned as a side effect, as if most cancer patients would not welcome some euphoria.)

The California study was conducted under protocols not calculated to yield good results. A participating researcher, oncologist Dr. Ivan Silverberg, noted, "The conditions were rigid, smoking times were prescribed; patients were not allowed to self-titrate their dose and were forced to smoke marijuana too quickly—and they could only smoke marijuana in a locked room. These restrictions seemed senseless to me. . . To smoke marijuana under the conditions established in the California state program essentially placed the patient in a hostile environment" [Silverberg[2]].

The California state study was the only one to find oral THC superior to smoked marijuana. Apparently, most subjects chose to take capsules rather than smoke cigarettes out of an aversion to smoking. Many subjects had no prior smoking experience. Others complained about the harsh quality of the smoke from the government's marijuana. Researchers reported,

"The characteristics of the NIDA cigarettes may have been a factor in discouraging further use by experienced marijuana smok-

---

[2] Affidavit of Ivan Silverberg, M.D., to DEA Administrative Law Judge Francis L. Young, reprinted in R.C. Randall, Ed. Marijuana, Medicine and the Law (Galen Press, 1988), p. 148.

ers. The cigarettes, even after proper storage, were dry and gave an acrid smoke. Their potency was noticeably low (1.2%-2.8%) at a time when street marijuana was increasing greatly in potency and availability.[3]"

Despite the promising findings about smoked marijuana in the state studies, official policy favored synthetic THC. In addition to being tainted by its illicit status, marijuana was criticized for being a natural plant whose ingredients and dosage were not rigorously controllable, whereas synthetic THC pills were regarded as more pharmaceutically pure and subject to precise regulation of dosage. In fact, as we have mentioned, the controllability of oral THC dosage was an illusion, given that subjects are better able to adjust their own doses with smoked marijuana through self-titration. Still, the Reagan administration encouraged the use of oral THC rather than marijuana, and in 1986 the FDA approved it for cancer chemotherapy under the name of Marinol.

Still, many patients find that smoked marijuana works better than legal synthetic alternatives. One obvious advantage of marijuana is that many chemotherapy patients are too sick to swallow a pill in the first place. Such patients find it much easier to inhale than to try to hold down a pill. In addition, of course, inhaled marijuana takes effect much faster, and its dosage is easier to control, making it less likely to produce unpleasant reactions.

Two other synthetic THC relatives, known as nabilone and levonantrodol, have been developed for cancer chemotherapy. Both are considerably less psychoactive than THC. Neither has won a large place in chemotherapy treatment, however.

A different, naturally occurring cannabinoid known as delta-8-THC was found to be completely effective in preventing vomit-

---

[3] California Research Advisory Panel, "Cannabis Therapeutic Research Program," Report to the California Legislature (Jan. 1989), p. 41.

ing in eight children who were cancer patients. Delta-8-THC is a close relative of delta-9-THC, with somewhat less psychoactive potency. Researchers observed "negligible" side effects in the children treated with delta-8-THC. Unfortunately, delta-8-THC is difficult to obtain, occurring only in trace quantities in natural marijuana as well as in Marinol, where it occurs as a by-product of chemical synthesis.

Over the years, the market has remained favorable to smoked cannabis as an anti-emetic. While demand for Marinol has languished, thousands of cancer patients and physicians have turned to marijuana—not that supplied by NIDA, of course, but good-quality, non-government grass. In some hospitals in California, cancer patients are allowed to smoke marijuana in designated areas or use smokeless vaporizers in their rooms. The judgment of oncologists is that marijuana is a useful medicine. In a survey of oncologists by Mark Kleiman and Rick Doblin at Harvard University, nearly half of all respondents said they would prescribe natural cannabis if it were legal to do so [Doblin[4]].

AIDS and HIV

Another common use of cannabis is in the treatment of nausea and appetite loss associated with AIDS. Some patients suffer severe weight and appetite loss, known as AIDS wasting syndrome, a condition whose impact on health and survival is severe. In Africa, wasting syndrome is a leading cause of death from AIDS, though it has become increasingly rare in the U.S. with the development of improved anti-viral therapy.

Many more patients suffer nausea from the drugs used to treat HIV and AIDS. Standard anti-retroviral treatments for HIV,

---

[4] Rick Doblin & Mark Kleiman, "Marihuana as Anti-emetic Medicine: A survey of Oncologists' Attitudes and Experiences," Journal of Clinical Oncology 9:1275-80 (1991).

such as AZT and 3TC, can cause major nausea. So can foscar-net, used to treat an HIV-related eye infection, cytomegalovirus retinitis. A major advance in HIV/AIDS therapy has been the introduction of protease inhibitors, which can help prolong pa-tients' lives indefinitely. Successful treatment typically requires following a complicated regime using a cocktail of drugs that can be extremely unpleasant and nauseating.

Many AIDS patients and doctors have found that marijuana helps them fight nausea, stimulate appetite and maintain their regimen. The results can be dramatic: some people with AIDS (PWAs) have reported weight gains as great as 40 or 50 pounds in a few weeks. A Stanford School of Medicine study found that HIV patients using medical marijuana were 3.3 times more likely to adhere to anti-retroviral therapy than non-users [De Jong[5]].

The benefits of oral THC have been proven in clinical testing of Marinol. An impressive 70% of HIV patients showed measur-able weight gain after treatment with Marinol. One fifth of the patients had to discontinue treatment because of adverse side ef-fects, which might have been lessened by the use of marijuana instead. In 1993, Marinol was approved by the FDA as safe and effective for treatment of AIDS-related wasting.

Marijuana is also useful for relieving other HIV-related com-plaints, including leg cramps, headaches, chronic fatigue, and pain. Many PWAs suffer from a painful condition known as peripheral neuropathy, characterized by stabbing or burning pains in the hands or feet. In a controlled, double-blind, study of 50 HIV patients, Dr. Donald Abrams of the University of California at San Francisco reported a 34% reduction in neu-ropathy pain among patients who smoked one NIDA marijuana

---

5 De Jong, Bourke C; et al, "Marijuana Use and its Association With Adherence to Antiret-roviral Therapy Among HIV-Infected Persons With Moderate to Severe Nausea," Journal of Acquired Immune Deficiency Syndrome 38:1 (2005).

cigarette three times a day [Abrams[6]]. Smoking the first cigarette reduced chronic pain ratings by a median of 72%.

Published in 2007, Dr. Abrams' study was the first U.S.-approved efficacy study of medical marijuana in nearly 20 years. Dr. Abrams had originally sought to study marijuana and AIDS wasting syndrome in 1994. Even though his proposal was FDA-approved, it was blocked by government bureaucrats, who refused to allow him access either to NIDA's own ample supplies of marijuana or to imported supplies from the Netherlands. Under pressure from the Drug Czar's office to resist medical marijuana research, NIDA reversed its long-standing policy of selling marijuana to any licensed researchers who requested it and mandated instead that they undergo a lengthy agency review. Eventually, Dr. Abrams was permitted to proceed with a small pilot study, on the condition that he not examine the efficacy, but only the safety of marijuana in HIV patients.

In 2003, he published the results under the title, "Short-Term Medical Cannabis Does Not Harm HIV+ Patients." [Abrams[7]]. The study found no harmful changes in HIV virus levels among patients who smoked marijuana. Instead, it found a 20% rise in T-cell counts, suggesting therapeutic benefits. Abrams noted that his findings contradicted results of previous, non-clinical studies, suggesting that smoked marijuana might suppress the immune system. The study also found a significant weight gain both from smoked marijuana and Marinol, although this was no longer a purpose of the study as revised by NIDA. Dr. Abrams went on to conduct his study on peripheral neuropathy under the auspices of California's Center for Medicinal Cannabis Research, the only

---

[6] Abrams, Donald; et al, "Cannabis in painful HIV-associated sensory neuropathy: a randomized placebo-controlled trial," Neurology 68:515-21 (2007).
[7] Abrams, Donald; et al, "Short-Term Effects of Cannabinoids in Patients with HIV-1 Infection: A Randomized, Placebo-Controlled Clinical Trial, Annals of Internal Medicine 139.4:258-266.

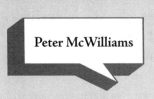

Peter McWilliams

"I use marijuana to treat the nausea caused by AIDS medications. Medical marijuana, for me, is a matter of life and death."

institution that has managed to secure access to NIDA's marijuana for medical research. In 2008 another CMCR study by Dr. Ronald Ellis confirmed Dr. Abrams' findings on the efficacy of smoked marijuna for neuropathic pain from HIV [Ellis[8]] Other CMCR studies are in the works.

Despite the government's resistance, marijuana has won widespread acceptance among AIDS patients and physicians. PWAs have played a prominent role in the medical marijuana movement. HIV patients accounted for some 80% of the 10,000 members of the first medical cannabis patients' group, Dennis Peron's San Francisco Cannabis Buyers' Club. A Canadian survey found that one in three HIV patients in Ontario used cannabis for appetite loss, nausea, vomiting, and sleeplessness [Furler[9]]. A survey of HIV patients in San Mateo, California, found that 52% used marijuana for nausea or appetite loss, 28% for pain, and 57% for anxiety and depression due to illness [Koopman[10]]. Researchers concluded that more HIV patients use cannabis for mental than for physical reasons.

One health concern connected with the use of marijuana for HIV patients is the risk of respiratory infections from smoking. Because of their compromised immune systems, PWAs are high-

---

8 Ellis R, et al, "Smoked Medicinal Cannabis for Neuropathic Pain in HIV: A Randomized, Crossover Trial," Neuropsychopharmacology, pub. online Aug. 6 2008.
9 Reported by Michelle Furler at Ontario HIV Treatment Network research conference, Nov. 26, 2003.
10 "More HIV patients use cannabis for mental than for physical reasons," IACM Bulletin, June 22, 2003.

ly susceptible to the life-threatening lung infection pneumocystis carinii pneumonia (PCP). Smoking is known to lower resistance to respiratory infections. In a recent Johns Hopkins University study of drug-using PWAs, those who smoked illicit drugs, including marijuana and cocaine, were twice as likely to contract PCP. The implications of the study are not entirely clear, since almost all of the subjects also smoked cigarettes. Still, PWAs should approach smoking with caution. The best alternatives to smoking are vaporizers and edible preparations.

One potential danger with smoked marijuana is contamination with bacteria and fungus spores, notably aspergillus fungus, which causes a lung disease that can be life-threatening to AIDS patients. Aspergillus infections, though rare, have been reported in cancer patients smoking marijuana for nausea. Patients should therefore take care not to smoke contaminated marijuana. See Chapter 6, "Preparation and Dosage Methods," for instructions on how to sterilize marijuana. Alternatively, many PWAs prefer to consume marijuana orally.

Critics have sometimes objected that the THC in marijuana has immunosuppressive properties that could be hazardous to AIDS patients. The fact that the FDA has approved Marinol for treatment of AIDS should indicate that this claim is a red herring. The immunosuppressive effects of cannabinoids are disputed, but appear to be at most marginal. Cannabis is better described as an "immunomodulator," tuning or balancing the response of the immune system by stimulating certain responses in some instances and suppressing them in others.

In any case, the particular immunosuppressive effects attributed to marijuana are not of a kind that should aggravate HIV infections. This is because the primary effect of HIV is the suppression of the production of the immune system's T-cells. Cannabinoids have no known adverse impact on T-cell counts. In fact, as mentioned above, one of Dr. Abrams' studies suggested that marijuana use actually boosts T-cell counts.

Epidemiological surveys of recreational users have found no evidence that marijuana increases susceptibility to AIDS, as charged by some anti-drug extremists. In fact, a San Francisco Men's Health Survey of 354 HIV-positive men found a decreased rate of progression to AIDS among marijuana users, although the difference was not statistically significant when adjusted for other factors, in particular the initial health of the different study populations. The Multicenter AIDS Cohort study examined 1,662 HIV-positive drug users, 89% of whom reported using marijuana [Kaslow[11]]. The study found no link between drug use and HIV disease progression or loss of CD4+ T-cells.

Hepatitis C

Many patients use marijuana to combat appetite- and weight-loss due to hepatitis C. Hepatitis C is a liver infection spread through blood, commonly found among intravenous drug users. Over time, it destroys the liver. Hepatitis patients are strongly advised to avoid alcohol because it aggravates liver damage. They are also strongly warned to avoid illicit drugs because of the close association between hepatitis C and drug abuse. Unlike other illicit drugs, however, marijuana may be helpful in treating hepatitis C. Because it is not injected, marijuana does not promote blood infections. Furthermore, many former drug abusers say that marijuana helps them avoid alcohol and other, more dangerous drugs such as heroin or cocaine.

---

[11] Kaslow RA, Blackwelder WC, Ostrow DG, et al, "No evidence for a role of alcohol or other psychoactive drugs in accelerating immunodeficiency in HIV-1-positive individuals: A report from the Multicenter AIDS Cohort Study," JAMA 261:3424-3429 (1989).

Despite this, the use of marijuana for hepatitis C remains controversial. Patients in liver transplant programs are commonly required to undergo urine testing to ensure that they are "drug-free." Because urine tests can detect marijuana for days after last use, this effectively precludes use of marijuana. Some hepatitis C patients have been kicked out of transplant programs and allowed to die on account of using medical marijuana.

Traditionalists defend this wanton discrimination on the assumption that marijuana users, like alcohol and other drug users, have a poor prognosis for surviving liver disease. The evidence for this is dubious. A couple of recent studies have reported a correlation between daily cannabis use and liver fibrosis in hepatitis C patients [Ishida and Hezode[12][13]]. However, the studies were not designed to show causality, and might reflect a tendency for patients with fibrosis to use more cannabis.

More convincingly, a study by researchers at the University of California at San Francisco and an Oakland substance abuse clinic found that marijuana use dramatically improved the effectiveness of hepatitis C therapy [Sylvestre[14]]. The study examined 71 patients taking two anti-viral drugs, ribavirin and interferon, with severe sided effects including nausea, loss of appetite, fatigue and depression. The drug regime was so grueling that many patients dropped out. After six months, 86% of the patients who used marijuana daily had successfully completed treatment, versus 59% of those who did not. Furthermore, 54% of the marijuana users showed a "sustained virological response" with no signs

---

[11] Ishida JH, et al., "Influence of cannabis use on severity of hepatitis C disease." Clin Gastroenterol Hepatol 6(1):69-75 (2008).

[13] Hezode C, et al., "Daily cannabis smoking as a risk factor for fibrosis progression in chronic hepatitis C," Abstract 68. European Association for the Study of the Liver 39th Annual Conference, 14-18 April 2004.

[14] Sylvestre D, et al., "Cannabis use improves retention and virological outcomes in patients treated for hepatitis C," European Journal of Gastroenterology and Hepatology, 18:1057-1063 (2006).

of the virus six months after treatment. Only 18% of those who did not use marijuana achieved this response. The investigators concluded that marijuana probably helped by improving appetite, reducing depression, and helping patients to better tolerate the treatment.

Morning Sickness and other Anti-Nauseant Uses

Some women use marijuana to treat the nausea of morning sickness, despite obvious concerns about fetal exposure during pregnancy. Though caution is always advisable in using drugs during pregnancy, marijuana doesn't appear to be especially dangerous to fetal health compared to other commonly used drugs, including tobacco, stimulants, and alcohol [Morgan & Zimmer[15]]. Experts now agree that marijuana does not cause birth defects. At worst, it may be associated with slightly lower birth weights. In any case, the risks of marijuana must be weighed against the benefits of relief from morning sickness, in which nausea can be so severe as to require hospitalization in some cases.

Cannabis is useful for numerous other conditions causing nausea, vomiting, and loss of appetite. These include various kinds of intestinal and kidney disease, adverse drug reactions, opiate addiction, and anorexia nervosa.

ANTI-CONVULSANT AND ANTI-SPASMODIC EFFECTS

One of the oldest established medicinal uses of cannabis is to treat muscle spasticity and convulsions. Cannabis was used to treat epilepsy as far back as medieval Arabia and sixteenth-century Southeast Asia. In 1839, when cannabis was first intro-

---

[15] Morgan & Zimmer, Marijuana Myths, Marijuana Facts, Chapter 13: Marijuana Use During Pregnancy.

duced to Western medicine by Dr. William O'Shaughnessy, it was applied to treat convulsions caused by tetanus (lockjaw) and hydrophobia (rabies), and then puerperal convulsions, chorea, and strychnine poisoning (with varying success).

Since then, cannabis has been found useful for a host of spasm-inducing disorders, including multiple sclerosis, spinal injuries, and many other conditions. Many of these diseases can be treated by a variety of prescription drugs, but not always satisfactorily, and often with debilitating, life-threatening, or otherwise intolerable side effects. Many patients report that they can reduce or eliminate their intake of toxic conventional medications and achieve better control of their complaints by smoking marijuana.

Though cannabinoids generally have anticonvulsant properties, they have also paradoxically been reported to precipitate muscle spasms in exceptional circumstances. As usual, this is most likely at higher doses. However, some animal studies have found that THC (though not CBD) at normal doses can excite nerve cell activity so as to promote convulsions. A few patients have been reported to exhibit myoclonic jerking or seizures after taking Marinol. Others say they are more apt to get leg cramps in bed after smoking marijuana.

According to Dr. Paul Consroe of the University of Arizona, there is reason to think that CBD may have distinctive therapeutic value as an anticonvulsant. Not only does CBD appear to lack the stimulant activity of THC; it may also help counteract THC's muscle-exciting tendencies [Consroe[16]]. For this reason, marijuana with high CBD may be preferable to Marinol in treating muscle spasticity.

In normal subjects, marijuana also produces adverse effects on

---

[16] Consroe P, and Snider S, "Therapeutic Potential of Cannabinoids in Neurological Disorders," Chapter 2 in Cannabinoids as Therapeutic Agents, Raphael Mechoulam, Ed., CRC Press (Boca Raton FL, 1986).

muscular coordination, a phenomenon familiar to anyone who has gotten too high. This deterioration, known as ataxia, is most apparent in tasks that are complicated or require prolonged attention. One test is to try to hold your hand or finger steady in the middle of a slightly larger hole without touching the edges. Another is to balance on one leg for thirty seconds. The effects of ataxia may to some extent counterbalance the benefits of cannabis for patients whose coordination is already impaired—for instance, by multiple sclerosis.

Spinal Cord Injuries, Paraplegia, and Quadriplegia

One of the most effective, yet under-publicized, uses of medical marijuana is for patients with spinal cord injuries. These patients often suffer severe chronic pain and muscle spasms, along with paralysis of the legs (paraplegia) or of both legs and arms (quadriplegia). Many find marijuana effectively relieves both spasticity and pain.

Spinal cord patients are commonly prescribed large doses of opiates, tranquilizers, and other debilitating and potentially dangerous drugs. Many find that they can dispense with these drugs altogether by using marijuana.

Preliminary studies by GW Pharmaceuticals have shown cannabis extracts to be effective in relieving pain and spasms from spinal cord injuries. A Swiss study of 25 patients with spinal cord injury reported that THC was effective in reducing spasticity in both oral and (ouch!) rectal doses [Hagenbach[17]]. Marijuana's usefulness is widely known both to patients and to physicians who specialize in pain control. In a survey of 43 spinal cord injury patients at VA hospitals, 56% reported smoking marijuana.

---

[17] Hagenbach U, et al, "The treatment of spasticity with Delta-(9)-tetrahydrocannabinol in persons with spinal cord injury," Spinal Cord 45:551–562 (2007).

Of that group, 88% reported that it reduced muscle spasms. Some VA hospitals allow marijuana to be smoked by paraplegics and quadriplegics in their wards.

Epilepsy

Epilepsy, which occurs in numerous forms, is characterized by the misfiring of overactive brain cells, causing a seizure. Epileptic seizures can take the form of bodily convulsions (violent spasms), loss of consciousness, loss of coordination, altered sensory states, and, in extreme cases, coma or death. Epilepsy can arise from various causes, including accidents, disease, and genetic factors. Conventional treatments, which include a variety of prescription anticonvulsant drugs, benefit many patients, but 20% to 30% cannot be adequately controlled.

Patients have found cannabis beneficial for two particular kinds of epilepsy. The first of these is grand mal epilepsy, which is characterized by violent bodily spasms, caused by abnormal brain cell misfiring on both sides of the brain. Numerous grand mal epileptics report that they are able to completely eliminate seizures by smoking marijuana, sometimes in conjunction with their regular medication and sometimes without it.

Cannabis may also be useful for complex partial seizure disorders, which are associated with damage to the frontal or temporal lobes of the cerebral cortex. These disorders appear in various forms: a loss of consciousness, muscular twitching, and so on. In general, they are not easily treatable. Again, certain patients find cannabis can suppress these problems. A survey of 308 epileptic patients reported that marijuana appeared to delay the first onset of complex partial seizures [Ellison[18]]. In a study by Cunha,

---

[18] Ellison WR, et al, "Complex partial seizure symptoms affected by marijuana abuse," Journal of Clinical Psychiatry 51:439 (1990).

half of temporal focus partial epileptics obtained complete relief of seizures with CBD at doses some 10 times greater than the amount typically found in a joint; however, other studies with CBD have not been so promising [Cunha[19]].

Cannabis is by no means a panacea for epilepsy. It is typically not useful for so-called petit mal or absence seizures. There is even evidence that CBD may counteract the efficacy of other drugs used for petit mal. Also, on at least one occasion, oral THC (at a dose of 20 mg) has precipitated a grand mal seizure in a patient with a previous history of epilepsy. Epileptics who are interested in trying cannabinoids should be careful about oral THC. Those who do use cannabinoids should be aware that they might become more susceptible to seizures when they withdraw from treatment.

Gastrointestinal Disorders

In recent years, medical marijuana has come into growing use to treat painful gastrointestinal disorders involving cramping and inflammation of the bowels. Among them are irritable bowel syndrome, colitis, and Crohn's disease. Patients report relief from symptoms such as chronic pain, cramping, inflammation, diarrhea and weight loss. Recent animal studies suggest that CB1 and CB2 receptors act to suppress gastrointestinal cramping, inflammation, acid reflux, and intestinal secretions. Doctors at the Mayo Clinic found that Marinol relaxed the colon and reduced stomach cramps after eating in a study of 52 volunteers [ACG[20]]. A survey of 18 Crohn's patients by Dr. Jeffrey Hergenrather of Sebastopol, California, reported improvements in pain, appetite, nausea, vomiting, fatigue, activity and depression. Relief has also been reported from a rare genetic disease called

---

[19] Cunha JM, et al, "Chronic administration of Cannabidiol to Healthy Volunteers and Epileptic Patients," Pharmacology 21:175-85 (1980).
[20] Press release by American College of Gastroenterology, October 23rd, 2006.

Peutz-Jeghers syndrome, which causes similar bowel complaints. In the nineteenth century, cannabis was used to treat cholera, in order to relieve both diarrhea and vomiting. Today, cholera is treated with other, modern therapies.

Menstrual disorders and labor pain

Many women find that marijuana relieves menstrual cramps or dysmenorrhea. This may result from the cannabinoids' suppression of prostaglandins. Dysmenorrhea was commonly treated with cannabis in the nineteenth century, and is said to have been the purpose for which Queen Victoria was prescribed cannabis by her personal physician, Dr. John Russell Reynolds. Many women find marijuana useful in treating other symptoms of premenstrual stress (PMS), such as tension, dysphoria and headaches. Cannabis has also been reported useful for endometriosis, an inflammation of the uterine lining.

Cannabis was traditionally used to ease labor distress during childbirth. This is the most ancient medical use of marijuana that is archaeologically confirmed. In a third-century tomb, Israeli archaeologists discovered the body of a girl who had apparently died in childbirth with traces of hashish at her bedside. Unfortunately, there has been absolutely no modern medical research on the efficacy of cannabis for childbirth.

Tourette's Syndrome

Tourette's syndrome (TS) is a mysterious, complex neuro-psychiatric disorder marked by facial and vocal tics, including involuntary verbal outbursts. The cause of TS is unknown. Its severity is variable, but its worst expression can be quite disabling. Con-

On Medical Marijuana Use for Chemotherapy

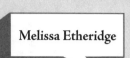

Melissa Etheridge

"[T]here's the drug that you take for the pain. But that constipates you. So, you have to take the constipation drug. But then that actually gives you diarrhea. So, you need a little diarrhea drug. Instead of taking five or six of the prescriptions, I decided to go a natural route and smoke marijuana."

"Medicinal marijuana—absolutely; every doctor I talked to...said that's the best thing to do…From the surgeons to the oncologists to the radiation. Every single one was, 'Oh, yeah. That's the best help for the effects of chemotherapy.'"

trolled studies by Dr. Kirsten Muller-Vahl at the Medical School of Hanover, Germany found that oral THC significantly improved symptoms in Tourette's patients, including reductions in tic severity and obsessive-compulsive behavior [Muller-Vahl[21]]. Similar effects have been observed with inhaled marijuana.

Other Movement and Muscle Spasm Disorders

Cannabis is helpful for numerous other movement disorders, some common and others too obscure to be listed here. Because of the government's hostility to medical marijuana research, there have been few human studies in this area. However, the following uses have been confirmed by anecdotal reports.

---

[21] Muller-Vahl K, et al, "Treatment of Tourette's Syndrome with Delta-9 THC: a randomized crossover trial," Pharmacopsychiatry 35:57-61 (2002).
Muller-Vahl K, et al, "Delta-9 THC is effective in the treatment of tics in Tourette's syndrome: a 6-week randomized trial," Journal of Clinical Psychiatry 64:459-65 (2003).

TABLE 1
Reported Effects of Marijuana Treatment on Features of Neurological Disorders Described in the 19th Century and Possible Contemporary Analogies to These Neurological Disorders

Disorders of the 19th century	Contemporary disorders	Effect of marijuana
Convulsions: recurrent, general, tonic, clonic	Tonic-clonic seizures generalized epilepsy	Benefit
Convulsions, petit mal	Absence seizures, generalized epilepsy	No effect
Spasms of torticollis and writer's cramp	Dystonic movements; spasmodic torticollis; writer's cramp	No effect
Rheumatic chorea generalized chorea effect	Choreic movements; Sydenham's chorea; Huntington's chorea	Benefit, no effect
Tremor of paralysis agitans	Resting tremor; Parkinson's disease	No effect
Tonic painful spasms; jerky movements of spinal effect sclerosis	Spasticity and ataxia; spinal cord injury; multiple sclerosis	Benefit, no effect
Pain of neuropathy, e.g. sciatica	Sustained pain; neuropathic pain	No effect
Pain of neuropathy, e.g., trigeminal neuralgia	Paroxysmal pain; neuropathic pain	Benefit
Migraine headache	Migraine headache	Benefit

© Dr. Consroe and Dr. Sandyk, CRC PRESS

Dystonia

Dystonia is a common kind of movement disorder characterized by painful tension and involuntary contractions in the muscles. There are anecdotal reports in the medical literature that marijuana and oral THC can be effective in treating dystonia [Chatterjee and Jabusch[22]]. It has been speculated that CBD or other

---

[22] Chatterjee A, et al, "A Dramatic response to inhaled cannabis in a woman with central

TABLE 2

Predicted Effects of (—)-Δ9-Tetrahydrocannabinol (THC) and Cannabidiol (CBD) on Contemporary Neurological Disorders Based on Their Reported Activity in Animal Models

Disorder or symptom	Animal model	Drug	Predicted Effect
Partial (simple and complex) seizures	Focal seizures	THC	Aggravate or benefit
		CBD	Benefit
Tonic-clonic seizures (grand mal)	Maximal generalized seizures	THC	Benefit
		CBD	Benefit
Absence seizures (petit mal)	Minimal generalized seizures	THC	No effect or aggravate
		CBD	No effect
Dystonia, Huntington's chorea, Tourette's syndrome, and tardive dyskinesia	Reserpine-induced hypokinesia	THC	Benefit
		CBD	Benefit
Parkinsonism: hypokinesia	Reserpine-induced hypokinesia	THC	Aggravate
		CBD	Aggravate
Dystonia	Inherited dystonia	CBD	Benefit
Huntington's chorea	L-Pyroglutamate-induced behavioral disturbance	CBD	Benefit
Spasticity	Polysynaptic and monosynaptic reflexes	THC	Benefit, or aggravate
		CBD	Benefit
Cerebellar ataxia	Cannabinoid-induced ataxia	THC	Aggravate
		CBD	No effect
Migraine headache	Nociception, edema and prostaglandins	THC	Benefit
		CBD	No effect

© Dr. Consroe and Dr. Sandyk, CRC PRESS

cannabinoids might moderate progression of dystonia, but clinical evidence is lacking.

---

thalamic pain and dystonia," Journal of Pain and Symptom Management 24.1:4-6 (2002). Jabusch HC, et al., "Delta-9 THC improves motor control in a patient with musician's dystonia," Movement Disorders 19.8:990-1, (2004).

TABLE 3

Reported Effects of Marijuana (MJ), (—)–Δ⁹–Tetrahydrocannabinol (THC) and Cannabidiol (CBD) on Contemporary Neurological Disorders

Disorder	Major symptom	Drug	Effect
Focal epilepsy	Partial (simple and partial complex) seizures	MJ CBD	Benefit Benefit or no effect
Generalized epilepsy	Tonic-clonic seizures (grand mal)	MJ THC Analog CBD	Benefit Benefit Benefit or no effect
Generalized epilepsy	Absence seizures (petit mal)		
Dystonias	Dystonia	CBD	Benefit
Huntington's disease	Chorea	CBD	No effect
Tourette's syndrome	Tics	MJ	Benefit
Tardive dyskinesia	Oro-buccal-lingual dyskinesia	MJ	No effect
Parkinson's disease	Resting tremor; rigidity hypokinesia	MJ CBD	No effect Aggravate
Multiple sclerosis and spinal cord injury	Spasticity; intention tremor; ataxia	MJ THC	Benefit Benefit
Neuropathic conditions	Sustained pain	CBD	No effect
Migraine	Pain and other symptoms	MJ	Benefit

© Dr. Consroe and Dr. Sandyk, CRC PRESS

Cerebral palsy

Some say that cannabis is helpful for cerebral palsy, a movement disorder caused by central nervous system injury during birth. Among them is Darrell Paulsen, a disabled rights activist from Minnesota, who says that cannabis controls his muscle spasms so well that he can use the restroom in minutes instead of hours. There have been no clinical studies of cannabis for cerebral palsy.

Choreas

This category of disorders is characterized by ceaseless, rapid, complex, jerky movements. In the nineteenth century, cannabis was used to treat Sydenham's chorea, a children's illness caused by rheumatic fever, which is now quite rare. More common today is Huntington's chorea, a progressive, degenerative disease of genetic origin, which claimed folk singer Woody Guthrie. There has been speculation, but no good evidence, that cannabis might be helpful in Huntington's; trials with CBD have shown mixed results [Consroe[23]].

Tardive dyskinesia

This disorder, which manifests itself in involuntary chewing and darting of the tongue, is an insidious side effect of the long-term use of antipsychotic drugs. Contrary to expectations, marijuana has yet to show evidence of clinical efficacy. On the other hand, it does not cause TD, as some critics have alleged.

As always, people with psychotic disorders should approach cannabis cautiously, since it may aggravate—as well as alleviate—such illnesses.

Parkinson's Disease

Parkinson's disease is a degenerative, progressive disorder, characterized by slow movement (hypokinesia), stiffness, and tremor. L-Dopa, the drug of choice for Parkinsonism, causes a movement disorder, dyskinesia, which might theoretically respond to cannabinoids. While some say that cannabis alleviates Parkinson-related symptoms, the evidence is unclear. Clinical studies

---

[23] Consroe P, et al, Controlled clinical trial of cannabidiol in Huntington's disease. Pharmacology, Biochemistry and Behavior. 40.3:701-8 (1991).

have been disappointing. A controlled clinical trial of 19 subjects by Dr. Camille Carroll at the University of Plymouth, England found that an oral cannabis extract had no effect one way or another on symptoms [Carroll[24]]. There is some evidence that prolonged usage of cannabis is needed to alleviate Parkinson's symptoms. A survey of 339 Parkinson's patients by researchers in Prague found that 46% of those who used cannabis reported that their symptoms were greatly relieved, but only after an average of 1.7 months of use. Most took cannabis orally [IACM[25]].

Black Widow Poisoning

The venom of the black widow spider causes severe, painful muscle cramps. Carol Miller, a California herbalist, says she found marijuana helpful in treating her husband for a black-widow bite. "His lower spine and upper body became wracked with horrible pain. The problem was getting him to smoke, because his jaw was locked up. A tincture would have worked better," she reports.

It is interesting that one of the earliest uses of cannabis in Western medicine was to treat lockjaw, or tetanus. Physicians reported mixed success with this treatment. Needless to say, anyone who comes down with tetanus, or has been bitten by a black widow, should seek immediate medical attention.

ANALGESIA (PAIN RELIEF)

Marijuana has been used to provide pain relief, or analgesia, for a wide variety of conditions, ranging from migraines and rheumatism to severe chronic pain caused by spine and nerve injuries,

---

[24] Carroll CB, et al, "Cannabis for Dyskinesia in Parkinson disease: a randomized double-blind crossover study," Neurology 63.7:1245-50 (2004).
[25] IACM Bulletin, 24 November 2002; original source: Reuters Health, 13 Nov. 2002.

cancer, and other illnesses. Two thousand years ago, the Chinese used high doses of cannabis to prepare patients for major surgery. The analgesic properties of cannabis were exploited in the nineteenth century to treat migraines, rheumatism, menstrual pains, and terminal illness. These uses declined with the development of the more effective opiates, such as morphine, which were stronger and more consistent in their effects, especially in the era before the discovery of THC (1964), when reliable methods for assessing the potency of cannabis medicines were not available.

Chronic Pain

Today, however, many patients find that cannabis is uniquely superior to prescription analgesics in controlling chronic pain. In fact, chronic pain constitutes the largest single use of medical marijuana. In Oregon, which maintains the largest state medical marijuana registry, 88% of the state's 14,831 patients report using marijuana for "severe pain" (including many who use it for multiple other complaints). In Dr. Mikuriya's practice, the largest single primary indication for medical cannabis, comprising 46% of all patients, was pain, followed by mood disorders (27%) and spasms and convulsions (9%) [Gieringer[26]].

Severe chronic pain is commonly treated with opioid narcotics – e.g., codeine, morphine, oxycodone (in Percocet®, Vicodin® and OxyContin®), and methadone–or other synthetic analgesics. The opiates are notoriously addictive and may become less effective as patients develop tolerance to them. In addition, many patients find themselves incapacitated by the stupefying and soporific effects of these drugs. Other, non-addictive synthetic analgesics are available, but they are often not strong enough. Some, such

[26] D. Gieringer, "Medical Use of Cannabis: Experience in California," Chapter 12 in Cannabis and Cannabinoids: Pharmacology, Toxicology, and Therapeutic Potential, F. Grotenhermen and E. Russo, Ed., (Haworth Press, Binghamton, NY 2002).

as the common over-the-counter analgesic acetaminophen (Tylenol®), which is also an ingredient in Percocet® and Vicodin®, carry a substantial risk of fatal liver damage in excess dosage.

Many patients find that by smoking marijuana they can completely eliminate potent drugs such as opiate narcotics. A good example is Bill, who suffered sciatic pain in the back and legs following spinal fusion surgery: "My doctors prescribed heavy doses of prescription painkillers, including morphine and methadone, after my operation. My legal medicine left me feeling heavily drugged, yet still in pain and unable to lead a tolerable life. I became suicidal. Then one of my doctors suggested I try marijuana. When I tried it, I discovered that it relieved the excruciating, sharp, electric pain I had been experiencing. Although I still experienced some dull, throbbing pain, my level of discomfort was now tolerable, with no 'drugged' or negative side effects. Marijuana turned out to be a godsend for me."

According to the nineteenth-century authority, Dr. James B. Mattison, cannabis often turned out to be an "efficient substitute for the poppy" in the treatment of patients addicted to opium, chloral, or cocaine. "Its power in this regard has sometimes surprised me," he reported.

Recent research has cast light on the analgesic action of cannabinoids. Studies have found that THC and other cannabinoids inhibit acute responses to pain stimuli. Cannabinoids appear most effective at relieving enhanced pain sensitivity (hyperalgesia) and chronic pain associated with nerve damage and inflammation. Cannabinoids act through the central nervous system via CB1 receptors in the brain and spinal cord as well as peripherally through direct action in the affected body tissues via CB2 and CB1 receptors.

Like opiates, cannabinoids block pain pathways in the central nervous system, but through a different neurochemical signaling system. Cannabis and opium therefore afford differing degrees of relief for different conditions. Some patients can completely replace opiates using cannabis; others find that they can significantly reduce their dependence on opiates. There is evidence that cannabis and opiates act synergistically to complement or magnify each other's analgesic effects.

Unlike opiates, cannabinoids may also act directly on injured tissues, specifically by alleviating inflammation around damaged nerves. Unlike opium, cannabis is distinctly effective for neuritis and neuropathy – pain caused by inflamed or damaged nerves. As we have seen, Dr. Abrams' study found smoked marijuana effective in relieving peripheral neuropathy due to HIV. Studies by GW Pharmaceuticals have found marijuana extracts effective against neuropathy from diabetes and a kind of pain found in MS patients known as allodynia, characterized by painful reaction to a normally innocuous stimulus, such as the brushing of clothing. Another study by GW Pharmaceuticals found that Sativex was effective against cancer pain in patients who were not responding to opiates. The same study failed to find benefits from a pure THC extract lacking the CBD in Sativex.

In general, CBD by itself does not appear to be useful for treating pure pain. In conjunction with THC, however, it may help alleviate pain indirectly by its sedative action or by relieving muscle spasms.

A few studies have suggested that cannabinoids might reduce sensitivity to pain that is artificially induced by heat, pinching, chemical irritation, and so on; but the results have not been consistent. A recent study by Dr. Mark Wallace for the California Center for Medicinal Cannabis Research found that smoked marijuana was helpful in relieving artificially induced pain, but only at moderate doses [Wallace[27]]. Excessive doses actually increased pain sensitivity. This is one of several studies indicating that cannabinoids lose therapeutic efficacy at excess doses.

It's impossible to list all the painful diseases for which marijuana has provided relief. Many are unusual diseases that do not respond to conventional medication, such as nail patellar syndrome (genetic underdevelopment of the nails or the kneecaps and other joints); spinal stenosis (squeezing of the spinal column); eosinophilia-myalgia syndrome (EMS—a disease caused by adulterated tryptophan); patellar chondromalacia (softening of the kneecaps, or "runner's knee"); and pseudohypoparathyroidism (characterized by profuse growth of spurs on the bones). Many involve intense bodily pain associated with skeletal disorders or damaged nerves.

Marijuana is a favorite drug among disabled veterans with war injuries and is surreptitiously recommended at some VA clinics for hard-to-treat pain and muscle spasms. THC is said to be especially useful for "phantom pain" from amputated limbs; causalgias, or pain felt in limbs whose nerves have been damaged; and neuralgias, characterized by intense pain extending along the nerves—in particular, trigeminal neuralgia (tic douloureux), which causes acute stabbing pain in the jaw.

Cannabis has also been used with success to treat the chronic pain of advanced cancer. A study at the University of Iowa Clinical Research Center found that oral THC in doses of 5 to 10 mg was nearly as effective as 60 mg of codeine for relieving pain in 36 terminal cancer patients, with effects lasting several hours [Noyes[28]]. At double doses, 20 mg THC was found to be even

---

[27] Wallace M, et al, "Dose-dependent Effects of Smoked Cannabis on Capsaicin-induced Pain and Hyperalgesia in Healthy Volunteers", Anesthesiology. 107(5):785-796, November 2007.

[28] Noyes RJ, et al, "The Analgesic Properties of Dealt-9-THC and Codeine," Clinical Pharmacology and Therapeutics 18:84-9 (1975).

stronger than 120 mg of codeine; however, subjects found this dose too sedative and mentally incapacitating for their comfort. Of course, the psychoactive effects of THC depend greatly on the context in which it is taken, and they're much more pleasant to some people than to others. All but one of the patients in the Iowa study had no earlier marijuana experience; this made them more sensitive to adverse psychoactive effects.

For some, the psychoactive effect of cannabis may itself be analgesic. A final-stage cancer patient named Gordon used cannabis in a remarkable regimen of self-treatment for an advanced, terminal lymphoma that had spread to his pancreas and bone marrow. Gordon followed a rigorous regime of diet, exercise, and meditation, without any drugs except marijuana, which he used to aid his meditation. According to Gordon, pot did not make the pain go away, but helped him "learn to move right through it," reaching an ecstatic state of "vibrating blissfulness, where I felt very, very good." With repeated experiences, he found that the pain diminished and "the ability of the pain to grab my attention was lost."

Gordon, who cultivated his own marijuana, says that he was able to develop a specific strain that was especially effective in minimizing extreme pain. He found it was possible to hybridize different strains of cannabis that could specifically address different kinds of disorders, such as insomnia, physical and emotional disorders, and so on. Unfortunately, Gordon's labors were destroyed by the drug police.

Migraine

Many patients report that marijuana is useful for treating migraine headaches. Migraine is a form of severe headache, often accompanied by nausea and vomiting, that lasts for hours and recurs chronically. Migraines are precipitated by the dilation of arteries in the brain. An estimated 20% of Americans, three quarters of them women, are afflicted by migraine.

During the nineteenth century, cannabis was considered to be the drug of choice for migraine. "Were its use limited to this alone, [the worth of cannabis] would be greater than most imagine," wrote Dr. J. B. Mattison in 1891 [Mattison[29]]. Today, patients are typically treated with aspirin, ergot derivatives, and a host of other medications, including opiates. As usual in medicine, these treatments do not always work. Many patients find that marijuana is more effective than conventional prescription drugs.

So far, little scientific research has been done on cannabis and migraine. A proposed study by Dr. Ethan Russo was denied approval by U.S. authorities. Another study is currently in progress in Europe. There is some evidence that THC (but not CBD) inhibits the release of serotonin from blood platelet cells, a likely causal factor in migraines. Marijuana also seems to alter blood flow in the cerebrum, but the clinical implications of this fact for migraine are unclear. One investigator reported three cases in which former long-term pot smokers began having migraines shortly after giving up marijuana. Two had been free of migraines during their years of smoking; the third had had occasional headaches that pot quickly relieved [El Mallakh[30]]. The author concluded that chronic marijuana use might suppress susceptibility to migraines.

Migraine attacks are often preceded by visual disturbances, weakness, dizziness, ringing in the ears, and other symptoms. Many patients report that they can avert a migraine attack by smoking a joint at the first warning of onset. Others take a small dosage daily

---

[29] Mattison JB, "Cannabis Indica as an Anodyne and Hypnotic," in Mikuriya T, ed. Marijuana Medical Papers: 1839-1972 Medi-Comp Press 1973.
30 El Mallakh RS, "Marijuana and migraine," Headache 27: 442 (1989).

to ward off attacks. Patients say inhaled marijuana is preferable to oral preparations such as Marinol in such situations, because quick treatment is necessary. (There is no evidence that CBD or other non-THC cannabinoids are helpful against migraines.)

Paradoxically, on rare occasions, marijuana has also been reported to precipitate migraine attacks.

ANTI-INFLAMMATION, IMMUNE SYSTEM MODULATION, AND NEUROPROTECTION

In addition to being an analgesic, marijuana has unique anti-inflammatory properties. This has been shown in numerous animal studies, as well as reports by many arthritis patients who find that it reduces the pain and inflammation in their joints. Chemically, the anti-inflammatory properties of cannabinoids may be linked to an increase in the production of glucocorticoid hormones, which are used to treat inflammation, and a decrease in the synthesis of prostaglandin, a hormone involved in inflammation, which is also suppressed by aspirin.

Experiments by E. A. Formukong of the University of London indicate that the non-psychoactive cannabinoids cannabigerol (CBG) and CBD are more effective anti-inflammatory agents than THC [Formukong[31]]. According to Dr. Mahmoud El-Sohly, cannabichromene (CBC) also has good anti-inflammatory effects. CBC is a non-psychoactive cannabinoid that has been found in high concentrations in certain strains of marijuana, particularly from South Africa. Significantly, anti-inflammatory properties have even been found in non-cannabinoid ingredients of marijuana: olivetol, cannflavin, and beta-caryophyllene, a fra-

---

31 Formukong, EA, et al, "Analgesic and Antiinflammatory Activity of Constituents of Cannabis L.," Inflammation 12.4:361-71 (1988).

grant terpenoid that acts on the CB2 receptor [Gertsch[32]].

Other experiments have shown that THC can inhibit the aggregation of the immune system's platelet cells, which are a principal cause of inflammation. This may be one of THC's supposed "immunosuppressant" effects. Certain types of inflammation can be understood as the product of an overactive immune system, which attacks the body's own tissues. As we have seen, THC acts on the body's CB-2 cannabinoid receptors, which are especially dense in immune system cells. Cannabinoids appear to have the effect of correcting over-active immune responses, in effect fine tuning or modulating the immune system. Such modulation can be useful in treating autoimmune diseases where the body's immune system runs amok and attacks its own cells. Examples of autoimmune diseases include rheumatoid arthritis, multiple sclerosis, diabetes, and many rare genetic conditions.

Rheumatism and Arthritis

Cannabis has long been used to treat rheumatism, arthritis, and related diseases. This was a classical use of cannabis in the nineteenth century, when it was said to be as effective as opium for severe rheumatism. Although it is no longer prescribed in modern orthodox medicine, it is widely used by patients, who report that it has unique benefits as a painkiller, antispasmodic, and anti-inflammatory agent.

Rheumatism includes various diseases marked by inflammation or degeneration of the joints, muscles, or connective tissue. Symptoms include pain, stiffness, loss of mobility, and inflammation of the joints. Severe cases can become completely debilitating. The first line of defense is typically aspirin for both pain

---

32 Gertsch, J et al., "Beta-caryophyllene is a dietary cannabinoid," Proceedings of the National Academy of Science, on-line June 23, 2008.

and inflammation; severe cases often require stronger drugs, such as opiates for pain and corticosteroids for inflammation. These have dangerous side effects when they are taken regularly.

Many patients find cannabis helps relieve the chronic pain of severe arthritis or rheumatism of the joints. In addition to its analgesic effects, cannabis can relieve the painful muscle spasms that often accompany rheumatic disease. Many patients find cannabis beneficial for fibromyalgia, a mysterious rheumatism-like disease characterized by widespread musculoskeletal pain, fatigue, and tender spots in the neck and back. David, who suffers fibromyalgia along with shingles (a painful disease caused by the chicken pox virus) and an injured leg, says marijuana "helps me to relax, dial into what's going on, break down the pain's control. . . . You can't make the pain go away," he says, "but you can learn to live with it." A recent study at the University of Heidelberg in Germany found oral THC helpful in reducing fibromyalgia pain by as much as two-thirds [Schey[33]].

Among the most severe forms of rheumatism is rheumatoid arthritis (RA), a progressive, degenerative disease that attacks the entire body. RA can become completely debilitating, causing deformation of the limbs and eventual death. Recent clinical studies of RA patients using Sativex have found that cannabis extracts can produce significant improvements in pain, sleep, and inflammation [Blake[34]]. There is even some evidence to suggest that cannabinoids can slow the progression of RA. In an animal study, investigators at London's Kennedy Institute of Rheumatology reported that treatment with CBD appeared to protect against joint damage and disease progression [Reuters[35]]. Similar results

---

33 Schley M, et al: "Delta-9-THC based monotherapy in fibromyalgia patients on experimentally induced pain, axon reflex flare, and pain relief." Current Medical Research and Opinion 22:1269-1276 (2006).

34 Blake DR, et al: Preliminary assessment of the efficacy, tolerability and safety of a cannabis medicine (Sativex) in the treatment of pain caused by rheumatoid arthritis, Rheumatology 45:50-52 (2006).

35 Research by Dr. Cornelia Weyand reported by Maggie Fox of Reuters, "Study May Force

have been observed with the synthetic cannabinoid HU-320.

One RA patient, Tom, who studied the preparation of canna-bis in cooking, found that marijuana helped relieve his inflam-mation when he took it in strong oral doses. He reported that oral ingestion was needed to achieve the desired effect because it is difficult to consume a sufficient dose through smoking. "It's much better eaten," said Tom. "Smoking gives muscle relaxation rather than pain relief." Tom's medical dose was 2 g, twice the standard recreational dose. Though this amount is likely to be incapacitating for normal daily functioning, Tom could take it at bedtime and wake up free of pain the next morning.

Neuroprotective Effects

"Scientific" information disseminated by governmental organiza-tions that promote and enforce cannabis prohibition would have you believe that marijuana is necessarily detrimental to your brain and nervous system. Yet nothing could be further from the truth. Although marijuana does temporarily stimulate the brain's natural 'forgetting faculty', this by no means implies that it is causing 'brain damage.' Recent scientific studies have shown that the cannabinoids in marijuana are actually neuroprotective, and can be used to prevent and treat toxic damage and inflamma-tion of the nerves. This is just one of many startling discoveries to emerge from the growing new field of cannabinoid medicine.

A growing body of research shows that cannabinoids can pro-tect nerve cells from death due to chemical stress caused by dis-

Re-Think on Rheumatoid Arthritis" Aug. 1, 2000. Research by Dr. Cornelia Weyand re-ported by Maggie Fox of Reuters, "Study May Force Re-Think on Rheumatoid Arthritis" Aug. 1, 2000.
For a summary of the state studies on marijuana for cancer chemotherapy, see Robert Ran-dall, ed., Marijuana, Medicine and the Law, Vol. 2 (Galen Press, Wash. DC) 1989

ease and injury. Studies show that cannabinoids protect against chemical oxidation, a leading suspect in many aging-related diseases. CBD in particular has been shown to be a potent anti-oxidant, like vitamins C and E [Mechoulam[36]]. THC and CBD can also protect against brain and nerve cell damage due to excessive glutamate. Glutamate is an excitatory neuro-transmitter in the central nervous system, which can build up to toxic levels in response to disease or injury. It is the same chemical found in the flavor enhancer monosodium glutamate (MSG), which, if taken in large amounts, can induce severe headaches and actually produce brain damage! A number of animal studies have found that cannabinoids protect nerve cells from glutamate toxicity. Thus cannabinoids can be neuroprotective, preventing nerve and brain damage and disease progression.

Multiple Sclerosis

Multiple sclerosis is a chronic, relapsing, progressive, neuro-degenerative disease in which the brain and the spinal cord nerves are damaged by the gradual destruction of myelin, the protective tissue that coats them. Its symptoms include painful muscle spasms, numbness, impaired vision, loss of coordination and balance (ataxia), tremors, and weakness, progressing to incapacitation and sometimes death. There is no known cure. According to the US National Multiple Sclerosis Society, about 200 people are diagnosed every week with the disease, typically ranging from 20 to 40 years of age.

Many MS patients find that marijuana helps relieve their symptoms, including spasticity, tremors, ataxia, depression, incontinence, and fatigue. Favorable effects have been confirmed in several

---

36 Mechoulam R, et al, "Cannabidiol – Recent Advances," Chemistry & Biodiversity 4:1678-92 (2007).

recent clinical studies using THC and cannabis extracts. Interest has been especially high in the U.K., where MS patients' groups have agitated for access to medical cannabis. Sativex, the oral cannabis spray developed in the U.K. by GW Pharmaceuticals, was first approved in Canada for treatment of MS pain. It has also shown promising results for spasticity and bladder control.

Numerous studies documenting the ability of cannabis to reduce MS-related symptoms including pain, muscle spasticity, depression, fatigue, and incontinence are now in the medical literature. A clinical study of 167 multiple sclerosis patients reported that Sativex relieved pain, spasticity, and bladder incontinence, with effects lasting for an extended period of treatment (mean duration 434 days) without requiring subjects to increase their dose [Wade[37]]. These results demonstrate that cannabis, unlike other drugs to treat pain and spasticity, does not rapidly induce tolerance. They also suggest that the cannabinoid therapy was actually slowing the disease progression since the same dose remained equally effective over the course of this extended study.

Remarkable benefits have been reported anecdotally as well. Noted Harvard Professor Dr. Lester Grinspoon has reported the case of Greg Paufler, who was severely debilitated by MS. Paufler found that marijuana restored his ability to walk, run, speak, and engage in sex, all of which he had lost [Grinspoon[38]]. Likewise, Dr. Mikuriya successfully maintained two MS patients with Marinol, supplemented by natural marijuana. One, a former aerospace engineer, suffered a relapse and became depressed and suicidal after losing his marijuana connection and being forced to rely on conventional therapies; he subsequently

---

37 Wade DT, et al, "Do cannabis-based medicinal extracts have general or specific effects on symptoms in multiple sclerosis? A double-blind, randomized, placebo-controlled study on 160 patients," Multiple Sclerosis 10:425-33 (2004).
38 Lester Grinspoon & James Bakalar, Marihuana, the Forbidden Medicine, pp.69-74 (Yale Univ. 1993).

recovered after regaining access to cannabis.

Recent studies suggest that cannabinoids can actually inhibit the progression of MS as well as mitigate its symptoms. This is because MS is a kind of autoimmune disorder, caused by a hyperactive immune system. As we have seen, THC appears to have mild immunosuppressive or immunomodulatory effects. Though these effects aren't important for most persons, they can benefit MS patients. Investigators at the Netherlands' Vrije University found that oral THC boosted immune function in MS patients, suggesting "disease modifying potential of cannabinoids for MS" [Killestein[39]]. Cannabinoids have also been found to have neuroprotective and anti-inflammatory effects on animals with MS-like conditions [Berrendero[40], Pryce[41]].

Follow-up studies are now being conducted on the long-term effects of cannabis on MS. As we shall see, there is reason to believe that cannabis is useful for other autoimmune diseases.

Amyotrophic Lateral Sclerosis

Amyotrophic lateral sclerosis (ALS), also known as Lou Gehrig's Disease, is a rapidly progressive, usually fatal, disorder characterized by the ongoing loss of motor neurons in the brain, spinal cord, and peripheral nervous system. The vast majority of ALS cases occur sporadically, with no known cause. ALS affects men more commonly than women and typically affects adults aged 40-60 years. Young males with ALS have the best prognosis and may have a longer life expectancy. A notable example is theoreti-

---

39 Killestein J, et al, "Immunomodulatory effects of orally administered cannabinoids in multiple sclerosis." Journal of Neuroimmunology 137:140-143 (2003).

40 Berrendero F, et al. "Changes in cannabinoid CB(1) receptors in striatal and cortical regions of rats with experimental allergic encephalomyelitis, an animal model of multiple sclerosis," Synapse 41(3):195-202 (Sep 2001).

41 Pryce G, et al, "Cannabinoids inhibit neurodegeneration in models of multiple sclerosis," Brain 126:2191-2201 (2003).

cal physicist Stephen Hawking, who was diagnosed with ALS in his early 20's and has now survived over four decades with the disease. Hawking still lectures all over the world, using a speech synthesizer activated by eye movement. Unfortunately the typical prognosis for ALS is grim with about half of all ALS patients dying within 2.5 years after the onset of symptoms. There are an estimated 30,000 Americans living with ALS; population studies indicate that the prevalence of ALS is increasing.

Studies suggest that excessive glutamate is involved in ALS. Serum, spinal fluid, and brain tissue of patients with ALS contain excessive levels of glutamate. As we have seen, cannabinoids can protect against glutamate toxicity. Animal studies have found that cannabinoids slow disease progression and prolong survival with ALS. One recent study showed that blocking the CB1 cannabinoid receptor extended the life span of mice with ALS [Bilsland[42]]. This suggests that some abnormality within our internal cannabinoid system may be part of the underlying disease mechanisms in ALS.

Based on these promising pre-clinical findings, some doctors (including a co-author of this book) are now recommending cannabis for their ALS patients [Carter[43]]. In addition to the neuroprotective effect, patients report that cannabis helps in treating symptoms of the disease, alleviating pain and muscle spasms, improving appetite, diminishing depression, and helping to manage sialorrhea (excessive drooling) by drying up saliva in the mouth. Indeed, in a large survey it was noted that ALS patients who were able to obtain cannabis found it preferable to prescription

---

42 Bilsland LG, et al, "Increasing cannabinoid levels by pharmacological and genetic manipulation delay disease progression in SOD1 mice," FASEB Journal 20:1003-5 (2006), cited in Armentano, "Emerging Clinical Applications for Cannabis and Cannabinoids," op cit.

43 Carter GT, Ugalde VO, "Medical marijuana: Emerging applications for the management of neurological disorders," Phys Med Rehabil Clin N Am 15.4:943-954 (2004); Carter GT, Rosen BS, "Marijuana in the management of amyotrophic lateral sclerosis," Am J Hosp Palliat Care 2001 18.4:264-70 (2001).

medication in managing their symptoms [Amtmann[44]]. However, this study also noted that the biggest reason ALS patients were not using cannabis was their inability to obtain it, either due to legal or financial reasons or lack of safe access.

Alzheimer's Disease

Alzheimer's disease (AD), or senile dementia, is a progressive, neurodegenerative disorder, like ALS and MS. Unlike ALS and MS, AD is characterized by a progressive deterioration of memory and overall cognitive functioning. Other symptoms of AD include aggressive behavior and agitation, depression, appetite loss, and, occasionally in advanced cases, difficulty walking. The damage due to Alzheimer's is caused by the formation of so-called amyloid plaques in the brain. There are only a couple of FDA-approved drugs to relieve symptoms of AD, and they don't improve longtime prognosis. AD patients typically survive from 8 to 10 years after diagnosis, eventually dying from brain damage.

For some while, cannabis has been used to treat the psychiatric side effects of Alzheimer's disease. Small-scale clinical trials have found that Marinol helps reduce anxiety, hostility, insomnia, and anorexia in Alzheimer's patients. A few doctors are currently recommending cannabis for these mental disturbances in Alzheimer's.

In addition, there is exciting new evidence to suggest that cannabinoids may actually help retard the progression of Alzheimer's. An animal tissue study at the Scripps Research Institute in California indicated that THC could inhibit the action of acetylcholinesterase, an enzyme thought to be responsible for amyloid plaques [Eubanks[45]]. The researchers concluded that THC

44 Amtmann D, Weydt P, Johnson KL, Jensen MP, Carter GT, "Survey of cannabis use in patients with amyotrophic lateral sclerosis," Am J Hosp Palliat Care 21.2:95-104 (2004).
45 Eubanks L, et al, "A molecular link between the active component of marijuana and Alzheimer's disease pathology," Molecular Pharmaceutics 3.6:773-7 (2006).

seemed "considerably superior" to FDA-approved drugs and might help treat both progression and symptoms of AD. A succession of other animal studies has found that CBD and some synthetic cannabinoids may prevent cell death and cognitive impairment due to AD. A recent review in the British Journal of Pharmacology concluded, "Cannabinoids offer a multi-faceted approach for the treatment of Alzheimer's disease by providing neuroprotection and reducing neuroinflammation, whilst simultaneously supporting the brain's intrinsic repair mechanisms" [Campbell[46]]. However, it must be noted that there have been no clinical studies to verify this in humans. At this point, there is no good reason to assume that medical marijuana is effective in treating the primary symptoms or progression of AD.

OTHER AUTOIMMUNE INFLAMMATORY DISEASES

Cannabis may be useful in treating many other inflammatory and autoimmune disorders. As we have seen, one example is multiple sclerosis, which is a kind of immune attack against the nerve cells' protective myelin coating.

Another example is diabetes mellitus, a disease characterized by excess blood sugar due to insufficient insulin production. Over time, it can cause damage to blood vessels, kidneys, and nerves and lead to blindness. Type 1 diabetes, also known as juvenile-onset or insulin-dependent diabetes, is typically caused by autoimmune damage to the pancreas. Type 2 diabetes, a less serious disease, is linked to genetic and dietary factors. Some animal studies have indicated that CBD can reduce the incidence of diabetes, lower inflammatory proteins in the blood, and protect against retinal degeneration that leads to blindness

---

46 Campbell VA & Gowran A, "Alzheimer's disease; taking the edge off with cannabinoids?", British Journal of Pharmacology Sep 10, 2007.

[Armentano[47]]. As we have seen, patients have also found marijuana effective in treating the pain of diabetic neuropathy.

A famous example is Myron Mower, a gravely ill diabetic who grew his own marijuana under California's medical marijuana law, Prop. 215, to help relieve severe nausea, appetite loss, and pain. Mower was arrested and charged with illegal cultivation after being interrogated by police in his hospital bed. In a landmark ruling, People v. Mower (2002), the California Supreme Court overturned his conviction, affirming that Prop. 215 gave him the same legal right to use marijuana as other prescription drugs.

While marijuana clearly provides symptomatic relief to many diabetics with appetite loss and neuropathy, scientific studies have yet to show whether it can also halt disease progression.

Pruritis and Skin Diseases

Cannabis may help relieve pruritis, severe itching caused by certain skin conditions as well as liver and kidney disease. GW Neff at the University of Miami reported that oral THC helped relieve pruritis in three patients with liver disease [Neff[48]]. Other studies have found encouraging results using topical skin applications of synthetic cannabinoids or endocannabinoids. This may have to do with the anti-inflammatory action of cannabinoids.

Some physicians have reported using cannabis to treat eczema and psoriasis, two common skin diseases associated with itching, inflammation, and autoimmune reactions. Topical applications are most commonly used for these and other skin irritations.

---

47 Armentano P, "Emerging Clinical Applications for Cannabis and Cannabinoids: A Review of the Recent Scientific Literature: 2000-2006," NORML Foundation Jan 31, 2007.
48 Neff GW, et al. "Preliminary observation with dronabinol in patients with intractable pruritis secondary to cholestatic liver disease." Am J Gastroenterology 97.8:2117-9 (2002).

Sickle Cell Anemia

Sickle cell is not an autoimmune disease, but rather a genetic blood condition that can produce severe chronic pain and inflammation. The pain is severe enough that patients are often treated with opiates. Many sickle cell patients have turned to cannabis as an alternative treatment. Among them is Sister Somayah, founder of a sickle-cell patient cooperative in Los Angeles, who won a jury acquittal under California's medical marijuana law after suffering repeated police raids for cultivation. A British survey of 86 sickle cell patients found that 36% were self-treating with cannabis to relieve pain, depression, and anxiety [Howard[49]].

Patients have reported cannabis to be beneficial for a host of other painful, debilitating, chronic autoimmune/inflammatory or genetic disorders, many of them obscure. Among those listed by Dr. Mikuriya are scleroderma, lupus, sarcoidosis, and mastocytosis. None of these applications has yet been investigated in controlled human studies; many are too rare even to contemplate FDA studies. Based on interviews with over 9,000 patients and 30 years of private practice, Dr. Mikuriya concluded that "cannabis appears to be a unique immunomodulator analgesic," useful in a wide variety of conditions.

PSYCHIATRIC AND MOOD DISORDERS

Marijuana's psychoactive effects have been variously described as euphoriant (inducing a sense of good feelings and well-being), sedative (mildly tranquilizing), anxiolytic (anxiety-reducing), and hypnotic (sleep-inducing). Such mood-altering effects can be medically useful in treating depression and other affective disorders. At the same time, however, marijuana can have negative

---

49 Howard J, Anie KA, Holdcroft A, Korn S, Davies SC, "Cannabis use in sickle cell disease: a questionnaire study," British Journal of Haematology 131.1:123-8 (2005).

effects, including paranoia, irritability, dysphoria (bad feelings), depression, depersonalization, and amotivation (loss of ambition). The interplay among these effects is complex and tricky, and their balance can alter from positive to negative in the same patient at various times. Because it is difficult for a person experiencing mood disorders to be objective, patients are strongly advised to consult a professional caregiver rather than to rely on self-medication for mood disorders.

Clinical Depression

Clinical depression is a serious illness, characterized by long-term, chronic, debilitating, sometimes suicidal feelings of sadness and low self-esteem. It should not be confused with simply feeling "down in the dumps," a state that is not properly treated with pharmaceuticals. Genuine clinical depression is regularly treated with a variety of prescription drugs: tricyclic antidepressants, monoamine oxidase (MAO) inhibitors, and, most recently, Prozac®. Bipolar depression, which is characterized by alternating high-energy "manic" and low-spirited "depressive" phases, is generally treated with lithium salts. Though most patients respond positively to prescription antidepressants, a minority do not, or cannot tolerate the side effects.

The mood-elevating properties of cannabis have been known since its first discovery as an intoxicant. The fabled Sufi credited with introducing hashish to Persia, Shaykh Haydar, is said to have made his monumental discovery after withdrawing into the fields in a state of depression. There he partook of the hemp plant, and "when he returned, his face radiated energy and joy, quite a contrast to his usual appearance as we knew him before." One of the first uses of cannabis in Western medicine, recommended by Dr. Jacques-Joseph Moreau de Tours, who spoke of

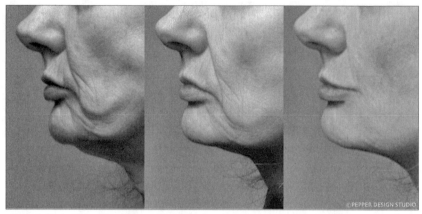

Onset of a Bipolar II depressive episode   *30 seconds after using cannabis*   *60 seconds after using cannabis*

Caroline, a Bipolar II, rapid cycler, treatment resistant patient: seventy-five percent of her life is experiencing extreme suicidal tendencies. "Prescription medication was ineffective at arresting my symptoms. Moments after use, cannabis relieves me of the physical and mental pain." *Photos: Larry Utley © Pepper Design Studio*

the "mental joy" of hashish intoxication, was for treatment of depression and melancholia. Depression is also listed as treatable by cannabis in early twentieth-century medical texts.

Later studies of depression had less positive results. In one double-blind test of THC versus placebo in eight depressed patients, not only did THC fail to relieve depression, but half of the patients experienced unpleasant anxiety and discomfort [Kotin[50]]. However, the artificial set and setting of this experiment may not have been conducive to good results.

More recent patient surveys indicate that marijuana is widely used to relieve depression. An Australian survey of medical cannabis users found that 56% used cannabis for depression [Swift[51]]. In many instances, depression is a secondary side effect of a more dangerous, life-threatening illness, such as cancer or HIV. Studies have found that patients using cannabis to treat MS, hepatitis C, HIV, Crohn's, sickle cell and other diseases also report reduced depression.

---

50 Kotin J, et al, "Delta-9-THC in depressed patients," Arch of Gen Psychiatry 28:345-8 (1973).
51 Swift W, et al, "Survey of Australians using cannabis for medical purposes," Harm Reduction Journal 2:18 (Oct 2005).

Many psychiatric patients who do not respond well to standard treatment find marijuana beneficial for depression. "The power of cannabis to fight depression is perhaps its most important property," says Dr. Mikuriya, a psychiatric specialist. Marijuana has been used successfully for both bipolar and regular clinical depression. Marinol has also been prescribed with success in such cases, although depression is an unlabeled use.

Like most of marijuana's psychoactive effects, euphoria does not occur consistently in all patients. Anti-euphoric, or dysphoric, reactions have been observed in numerous studies, especially among older patients who are not accustomed to mood-altering drugs. Individual users may also experience differing effects according to their own moods, expectations, and set and setting. When taken at the wrong time or in the wrong frame of mind, marijuana can provoke negative brooding.

An animal study by investigators at McGill University and the University of Montreal suggested that marijuana is effective against depression only in moderate doses, while long-term heavy use makes depression worse [Canadian Press[52]]. Researchers found that low doses of cannabis increased brain levels of serotonin, a neurotransmitter associated with positive mood, in laboratory rats. High doses depleted serotonin levels. "Our research shows that excessive cannabis use in people with depression poses a high risk of psychosis," concluded researcher Dr. Gabriella Gobbi.

Coincidentally, surveys have indicated that marijuana (and other drug) use, particularly among adolescents, is a risk factor in depression and other mental disorders. An Australian study by Michael Lynskey examined 277 pairs of twins, one of whom had used cannabis in childhood and the other of whom had

---

52 Reported by Sidhartha Banerjee, "Cannabis shows anti-depression benefits, but too much has reverse effect," The Canadian Press, Oct 23, 2005.

not [Lynskey[53]]. Those who used cannabis were found to have a 1.3 to 3.4 times greater risk of major depression and suicidal thoughts in later life. Another, 10-year study by the Max Planck in Germany found that the onset of cannabis use after age 14 to 17 was associated with depression, anxiety, and bipolar disorders [Wittchen[54]]. Given these studies, it is difficult to tell whether cannabis was actually a cause of depression, or was rather a response to it. In any case, the evidence militates for caution in exposing adolescents to marijuana.

In general, studies have shown that persons with mental disorders such as depression, anxiety and schizophrenia are more apt to use tobacco, alcohol, cannabis and other drugs. The question remains to what extent cannabis may exacerbate their problems, and to what extent it may be a valid form of self-treatment. A study of 119 marijuana-dependent psychiatric patients by New York researchers M. Arendt, et al, found that those with lifetime depression experienced more adverse symptoms, including depression, sadness, anxiety and paranoia, while under the influence of cannabis [Arendt[55]]. On the other hand, an Internet survey of 4400 adults by researchers at the University of Southern California found that marijuana users reported less depressed mood and more positive affect than non-users [Denson[56]].

In the Alice-in-Wonderland logic of drug bureaucrats, euphoria or elevated mood has sometimes been listed as an "adverse reaction" of marijuana. Of course, it's possible that some sullen

---

53 Reuters Health of 8 October 2004; Lynskey MT, et al, "Major depressive disorder, suicidal ideation, and suicide attempt in twins discordant for cannabis dependence and early-onset cannabis use," Arch Gen Psychiatry 61.10:1026-32 (2004).

54 Wittchen HU, et al, "Cannabis use and cannabis use disorders and their relationship to mental disorders: A 10-year prospective-longitudinal community study in adolescents," Drug and Alcohol Dependence 88, Supp 1:S60-70 (2007).

55 Arendt M, et al, "Testing the self-medication hypothesis of depression and aggression in cannabis-dependent subjects," Psychological Medicine 37:1-11 (2007).

56 Denson T and Earleywine M, "Decreased depression in marijuana users," *Addictive Behaviors*, 31:738-42 (2006).

or puritanical patients find euphoria disconcerting, but it's more likely that drug prohibitionists are upset that others find happiness in breaking the law.

As noted by the medieval Arab/Persian author of the Mukzunul-Udwieh, hemp drugs can have contrary stimulant and sedative effects: "They at first exhilarate the spirits, cause cheerfulness, excite the imagination into the most rapturous ideas, produce thirst, increase appetite, excite concupiscence. Afterward the sedative effects begin to preside, the spirits sink, the vision darkens and weakens; and madness, melancholy, fearfulness, dropsy, and such like distempers are the sequel."

Anxiety

Cannabis is often said to have calming and anxiety-reducing effects. Medically, it is used for many of the same problems as minor tranquilizers such as the benzodiazepines Librium® and Valium®, including convulsive-movement disorders, chronic pain, and so on. Certain patients feel that cannabis is superior to the benzodiazepines and other sedatives because it produces less dulling of mental acuity, although most users have the opposite impression, that cannabis is more apt to cause mental confusion.

Contrary to the popular image of marijuana as producing a "laidback" state, it can also aggravate anxiety. This can be seen in the well-known phenomenon of "panic reactions," which often trouble inexperienced users, especially at high levels of THC. Although panic reactions quickly fade with the effects of the drug, they can be frightening enough for some users that they seek medical help. In milder cases, users may simply be discomfited by heightened paranoia, self-consciousness, and anxiety. Panic reactions are sufficiently common that they have been mentioned in medical studies as a major impediment to medical use of cannabis. One aggravating factor here, as we have mentioned, is that the set and setting of medical studies tend to inspire nervousness rather than relaxation.

Experienced marijuana users appear to be less prone to panic attacks than inexperienced users. (Of course, one reason for this could be that persons who suffer panic reactions are less inclined to become regular users in the first place.) A study of 17 subjects by Mathew and Wilson at Duke University found that marijuana smoking increased anxiety in inexperienced users, but decreased it in experienced ones [Mathew & Wilson[57]]. Inexperienced users also reported increased depression. The authors related this to differences in cerebral blood flow in the two groups; unlike the experienced users, inexperienced users appeared to suffer a decrease in blood flow in the brain, perhaps caused by anxiety.

Other evidence suggests that the anxiety-enhancing effects of marijuana result mainly from THC and can be counteracted by CBD. Animal studies have generally found CBD to have anxiolytic (anxiety-dissolving) and antipsychotic effects. A study by A. W. Zuardi found that eight subjects given pure THC consistently felt more "discontented," "withdrawn," "troubled," "muzzy," "incompetent," "feeble," and "drowsy" [Zuardi[58]]. When given CBD, they were apt to feel more "alert," "quick-witted," "clearminded," "tranquil," and "gregarious." The combination of THC and CBD yielded intermediate effects. All this indicates that marijuana with CBD may be preferable to Marinol for dealing with anxiety. This has been born out in studies by GW Pharmaceuticals, which have found fewer adverse psychiatric effects using Sativex, which contains 50% CBD, than using pure THC.

---

57 Mathew and Wilson in: Murphy L, Bartke A, Eds. Marijuana/Cannabinoids. Neurobiology and Neurophysiology. Boca Raton, CRC Press, 1992, pp. 349-50.
58 Zuardi AW, et al, "Action of cannabidiol on the anxiety and other effects produced by delta-9-THC in normal subjects," Psychopharmacology 76:245-50 (1982).

Obviously, considerable caution must be used in recommending marijuana to patients with serious mental disturbances. Studies in Sweden, New Zealand, the Netherlands and Israel have found that youthful cannabis use is associated with a higher risk of schizophrenia. Though some critics have gone so far as to charge that marijuana actually causes schizophrenia, no increase in the rate of schizophrenia has been observed in the general population since marijuana became popular in the 1960s. However, the evidence indicates that heavy marijuana use in adolescents with a predisposition to schizophrenia can precipitate or aggravate symptoms. In short, while marijuana does not cause schizophrenia in healthy persons, it may make preexisting mental problems worse.

On the other hand, there is evidence that recreational use of cannabis may have a sedative effect on many mental patients. A survey of 79 psychotics by Richard Warner, et al found that those who used marijuana recreationally tended to report less anxiety, depression, insomnia, and physical discomfort [Warner[59]]. Relatively few experienced adverse effects such as paranoia and hallucinations. In contrast, most patients who drank alcohol reported that it aggravated their problems. The researchers concluded that marijuana might have a "useful, calming effect" in some patients.

In certain cases, cannabis may be helpful for schizophrenics. A study at the Berlin University of Medicine surprisingly found that among schizophrenics regular cannabis use was associated with improved cognition on certain tests [Jockers-Scherubl[60]]. The association was most pronounced among those who had started using before the age of 17. In contrast, cannabis use was

59 Warner R, et al, "Substance Use Among the Mentally Ill : prevalence, reasons for use, and effects on illness," American Journal of Orthopsychiatry 64.1:30-9 (1994).
60 Jockers-Scherübl MC, et al, "Cannabis induces different cognitive changes in schizophrenic patients and in healthy controls," Progress in Neuro-Psychopharmacology and Biological Psychiatry 31.5:1054-1063 (2007).

associated with poorer scores among non-schizophrenics. Yet another recent study found that cannabis use was associated with improved cognitive functioning in males with schizophrenia/schizoaffective disorder [Coulston[61]]. Those with more frequent and recent cannabis use scored better on tests of attention, processing speed and executive function – exactly the opposite of what would be expected in normal subjects. This suggests that some schizophrenics may have legitimate reason to treat themselves with cannabis.

Post-Traumatic Stress Disorder (PTSD)

Many patients find marijuana especially useful for alleviating post-traumatic stress disorder. PTSD is a psychiatric condition afflicting thousands of war veterans, and accident and crime victims who have undergone violent trauma. Victims experience enduring and often disabling depression, sleeplessness, anxiety, mood swings, fatigue, and irritability, as well as chronic pain and other discomforts stemming from their trauma.

Physicians in California's Society of Cannabis Clinicians treat many PTSD patients with cannabis. Dr. Mikuriya reported that 8% of his 9,000 patients have primary diagnoses for PTSD. Sleep deficit, fatigue and physical pain are symptoms commonly alleviated by cannabis.

> "Based on both safety and efficacy, cannabis should be considered first in the treatment of post-traumatic stress disorder," said Dr. Mikuriya. "As part of a restorative program with exercise, diet, and psychotherapy, it should be substituted for 'mainstream' anti-depressants, sedatives, muscle relaxants, tricyclics, etc. "

---

61 Coulston CM, Perdices M, Tennant CC, "The neuropsychological correlates of cannabis use in schizophrenia: Lifetime abuse/dependence, frequency of use, and recency of use." Schizophr Res 96.1-3:169-184 (2007).

"PTSD often involves irritability and inability to concentrate, which is aggravated by sleep deficit. Cannabis use enhances the quality of sleep through modulation of emotional reactivity. It eases the triggered flashbacks and accompanying emotional reactions, including nightmares. The importance of restoring circadian rhythm of sleep cannot be overestimated in the management of PTSD. Avoidance of alcohol is important in large part because of the adverse effects on sleep."

U.S. Army doctors, for whom cannabis is taboo, commonly prescribe veterans with PTSD anti-depressants, anti-convulsants, anti-psychotics, tranquilizers, and a host of other medications. Many report that marijuana works better than all their other prescriptions.

The Israeli army has indicated interest in testing THC to treat PTSD at the suggestion of pioneering cannabinoid researcher Dr. Raphael Mechoulam. Mechoulam hypothesizes that THC can relieve flashbacks of traumatic battle incidents by helping suppress unwanted memories. Animal studies by Giovanni Marsicano indicate that the endogenous cannabinoid system plays a role in extinguishing aversive memories as well as phobias and some kinds of pain [Marsicano[62]].

Attention Deficit Hyperactivity Disorder (ADHD)

Attention deficit hyperactivity disorder is a neurological disorder commonly diagnosed in children, with symptoms usually persisting into adulthood. Symptoms include difficulty in concentrating (inattention), difficulty in organizing and completing tasks, especially those that are repetitive, boring or difficult, and

---

62 Marsicano G, et al, "The endogenous cannabinoid system controls extinction of aversive memories," Nature 418.6897:530-534 (2002).

impulsiveness or hyperactivity, especially in children. In some cases the component of hyperactivity is lacking and the disease is referred to simply as attention deficit disorder (ADD). There is some dispute as to whether ADD is truly a disease or simply a variant of normal behavior, but extreme cases of ADHD can involve pathologically disruptive behavior. Some 3% to 7% of all children are thought to have ADHD or ADD; 70% of them show symptoms into adulthood.

Children with severe ADHD are commonly treated with psychoactive drugs. Paradoxically, the most popular drugs are stimulants such as amphetamines or Ritalin®, which regularly excite and stimulate normal people but help hyperactive children to stay focused.

In light of this paradox, it is perhaps less surprising that some pediatricians have reported beneficial effects with cannabis. Despite the fact that most people find that cannabis decreases their powers of attention, many people with ADD say it helps them focus. The use of marijuana for ADD is highly controversial, and there have been no scientific studies to validate it.

Nonetheless, benefits have been observed in some ADD patients. Dr. Claudia Jensen, a pediatrician from Ventura County, California, reported in Congressional testimony that cannabis was uniquely beneficial for two of her young ADD patients who had not been helped by other drugs [Jenson[63]]. For minors, Jensen first recommended Marinol. Only if that didn't work did she recommend marijuana, in the form of brownies or other edibles. (Use of smoked marijuana near school campuses poses obvious problems.) The use of cannabis by teenagers with ADD flies in the face of conventional wisdom, which assumes that marijuana is a step down the road to emotional withdrawal, disaffection,

---

63 Dr.Claudia Jensen, testimony to US. House Government Reform Subcommittee on Criminal Justice, Drug Policy and Human Resources, April 1, 2004.

amotivation, and stunted emotional growth.

Still, dramatic cases have been reported, such as that of young Jeffrey, whose story is told by his mother, Debbie Jeffries, in "Jeffrey's Journey."[64] At an early age, Jeffrey exhibited severe behavioral problems, including violent tantrums, aggression, hostility, and obsessive-compulsive behavior. He failed to respond to treatment with amphetamines and a pharmacopoeia of other mood-altering drugs. In desperation, his mother decided to try giving him cannabis, using edibles and capsules of organic marijuana prepared by the Wo/Men's Alliance for Medical Marijuana (WAMM) in Santa Cruz.

"Six months later, my eight-year old son wasn't angry with the world," Jeffries writes, "He was actually learning how to have fun, and for the first time ever, his outbursts had diminished enough so that he was capable of benefiting from psychological and behavioral counseling." Despite Prop. 215, Jeffries had to fight court battles with child protective services and school officials to continue treating her son. Then, on September 5, 2002, DEA agents raided WAMM's garden, cutting off Jeffrey's supply of marijuana. Without his medicine, Jeffrey relapsed. WAMM tried to reformulate his medicine using other strains of cannabis, but they didn't work as well. Eventually, his mother gave up, halted the cannabis treatment, and sent Jeffrey to a residential program. "Medical marijuana had given Jeffrey two years to grow and mature," his mother writes, "It is impossible to know what path his therapy would have followed if his treatment had not been disrupted by the federal government."

While Jeffrey represents an extreme, it is unclear how much patients with milder ADD benefit from marijuana. There exists an extensive drug abuse literature showing that adolescent

---

64 Quick American Publications 2005.

marijuana use is correlated with a constellation of mental health problems, including ADD, depression, low self-esteem, lack of motivation, poor school performance, and so forth. The popular interpretation by drug abuse experts is that marijuana use naturally aggravates such problems. An alternative interpretation is that adolescents may be—at least in certain instances—self-treating their underlying emotional problems with marijuana.

Dr. Thomas O'Connell, a cannabis practitioner in California who has painstakingly interviewed over 4,000 patients, has proposed this unorthodox view. Dr. O'Connell reports that his patients are using marijuana for a variety of mood disorders, especially stress, anxiety, dysphoria, panic attacks, depression, and insomnia. Some 15% of Dr. O'Connell's patients have ADD; 20-30% have bipolar disorder; and 10% report drinking problems. The vast majority also had prior experience with drugs beginning from adolescence, participating in the explosion in youthful drug use that began with the Baby Boom generation. Virtually all began using alcohol and marijuana before age 18 for non-medical reasons; 96% had tried tobacco; over 75% had experimented with mushrooms or other psychedelics, and over 67% had tried other illegal drugs. The great majority had an absent, distant, or disabled father; and most suffered low self-esteem, insecurity, and related psychological complaints. In short, Dr. O'Connell's patient population closely resembles the standard picture of marijuana users in the drug abuse literature. The difference is that whereas the standard literature interprets their marijuana use as drug abuse, Dr. O'Connell views it as self-medication:

"Anecdotal evidence from repeated clinical contacts, and other data gathered incidentally over five years of experience with this population suggests that, except for very modest alcohol consumption and obligatory (addictive) use of tobacco by those trying to quit, cannabis is the only drug used past the age of twenty-five by most. Indeed, their total drug histories suggest that by competing successfully with other, potentially more harmful agents, cannabis may have actually been protective.... For the majority, cannabis can be seen as an effective anxiolytic/antidepressant, performing as well or better than many currently available pharmaceutical agents prescribed for the same symptoms" [O'Connell[65]].

An accurate evaluation of these claims would require rigorous, controlled studies, in which subjects were observed both with and without marijuana to see how their symptoms responded. In the absence of such studies, the question remains open.

One thing should be noted, however: not all emotionally disturbed marijuana users are self-medicating. In a survey of cannabis-dependent users, Arendt, et al found that those with lifetime depression used marijuana for the purpose of getting high, not medication, and actually suffered worse depression, anxiety and paranoia while under the influence [Arendt[66]]. Those who had a history of violence were more likely to use marijuana for medical reasons in order to help relax and decrease aggression, but nonetheless manifested worse aggression when high. Marijuana is thus not always a solution for mood disorders, even for those who think it is. Patients with emotional disorders are strongly advised to follow professional counseling, not rely only on self-medication.

Chronic Fatigue Syndrome

Another anecdotal use of marijuana is for chronic fatigue syndrome (CFS), a mysterious illness of unknown etiology. Symptoms of CFS include debilitating fatigue, headaches, depression,

---

65 O'Connell T & Bou-Matar CB, "Long time marijuana users seeking medical cannabis in California (2001-2007): demographics, social characteristics, patterns of cannabis and other drug use of 4117 applicants," Harm Reduction Journal 4:16 (2007).
66 Arendt M, et al, "Testing the self-medication hypothesis of depression and aggression in cannabis-dependent subjects," Psychological Medicine 37:934-45 (2007).

muscle weakness, and other symptoms. Some CFS patients report that marijuana makes them feel better. Unfortunately, there have been no medical studies of this treatment.

Some enthusiasts claim to use marijuana for "stress." However, this is not a recognized medical indication for mood-altering drugs. Stress is not an internal mental disorder, but rather the effect of external pressures from everyday life. In contrast, tranquilizers are generally reserved for what are called "severe anxiety disorders," involving an inherent constitutional problem. Mood-altering drugs are not medically recommended as a way of coping with reality; on the contrary, such use is generally condemned by orthodox medicine. A widely deplored evil of cannabis abuse is its ability to encourage escapism and discourage users from dealing with their problems. This can be seen in the so-called amotivational syndrome, a tendency for users to disengage from the real world. Critics of marijuana may therefore condemn "stress reduction" as an excuse for recreational escapism. On the other hand, it is commonly accepted for Americans to drink alcohol after work in order to relax and relieve stress.

Insomnia

Many patients find that marijuana helps them sleep better. In the nineteenth century, cannabis was widely recognized as an effective hypnotic. Dr. J. R. Reynolds strongly recommended it for "senile insomnia." Tales of early hashish explorers are filled with accounts of dreams, torpor, and immobility, aggravated no doubt by heavy doses. In fact, overdoses of cannabis are known to make people pass out.

The hypnotic (sleep-inducing) properties of cannabis are of special value to chronic pain patients, many of whom rely on it for a good night's sleep. Quite a few healthy people also take a toke or two every night before bedtime to help them get to sleep. Medical studies have found that both THC and CBD by themselves help improve sleep.

Like other effects of marijuana, sleepiness is not a consistent effect. In fact, many users find that marijuana keeps them awake. In general, as we have mentioned, cannabis tends to be most exciting in the first hour or so after smoking, then gradually becomes more sedative.

In some instances, marijuana may suppress dreaming. Studies of sleeping subjects have shown that THC tends to suppress rapid-eye-movement (REM) sleep, during which dreams occur. These effects are most apparent at very high doses, and may decline with chronic use. We know of a Freudian psychotherapist who complains that her pot-smoking patients don't have enough dreams to report.

Former heavy users sometimes report insomnia and vivid dreams after giving up marijuana. These are withdrawal effects that subside after a few days or weeks. Some long-term pot smokers who believe they need marijuana to go to sleep may in fact only be suffering from withdrawal effects due to their heavy usage. In order to properly gauge the effects of marijuana, it's advisable for heavy users to abstain for a month or two to reach a THC-free baseline.

HARM REDUCTION SUBSTITUTE FOR ALCOHOLISM AND DRUG DEPENDENCY

Cannabis may provide a safer substitute for other, more harmful drugs, both recreational and medical. As we have seen, many patients find that marijuana can eliminate their dependence on potent prescription drugs, such as opiates, anti-depressants, anti-inflammatory agents, and so on, many of which have dangerous side effects when used regularly.

In addition, many ex-alcoholics, tobacco smokers and other drug addicts say they have been able to kick their habits by using marijuana as a substitute. Because marijuana is not toxic and less debilitating than heavy alcohol or hard-drug abuse, this is typically a healthy development. Unlike marijuana, excessive alcohol can be toxic to the liver, the brain, and the digestive and circulatory systems; it can also be physically addicting, producing life-threatening withdrawal symptoms in some cases.

Many alcoholics say that they have reestablished control of their lives by giving up alcohol for marijuana. The singer Bing Crosby, who had alcoholic tendencies, turned towards marijuana, and advised his son to do likewise. Benefits of marijuana substitution include avoidance of binge-drinking blackouts and hangovers, reduced depression, improved eating habits, and reduced hostility and violence toward others. A few ex-junkies report similar benefits from marijuana as a replacement for opiates.

Marijuana has sometimes been proposed as a treatment for addiction withdrawal symptoms. There is some evidence from animal studies that cannabinoids can reduce the effects of opiate withdrawal [Yamaguchi[67]]. In the nineteenth century, cannabis was tried in the treatment of delirium tremens, the shaking and convulsions associated with alcohol withdrawal; however, the results were not especially good. In general, marijuana appears to be less useful for withdrawal than as an outright replacement for other drugs.

Tobacco addicts have sometimes been known to substitute marijuana for cigarettes. The benefits of substitution are more doubt-

67 Yamaguchi T, et al, "Endogenous cannabinoid, 2-arachidnoylglycerol, attenuates naloxone-precipitated withdrawal signs in morphine-dependent mice," Brain Research, 909 (1-2):121-6 (2001).

ful in this case. Puff for puff, marijuana smoke delivers as many toxins as cigarette smoke, and its psychoactive effects are more impairing, if less habit-forming. Some nicotine addicts have successfully used marijuana to wean themselves from the cigarette habit. The joint provides oral satisfaction, a "smoke fix" for the lungs, and a sense of relaxation that can alleviate the craving for cigarettes. Once the nicotine addiction ends, smokers can work on tapering off the marijuana. One tobacco smoker reported using joints of "trim" — leaves removed during cleaning and processing — whenever he was tempted to smoke. The trim wasn't very potent but it satisfied his smoke craving.

Cannabis substitution is by no means accepted by the drug treatment establishment, which in recent years has become committed to the goal of total drug abstinence as preached in the twelve-step recovery programs such as Alcoholics Anonymous. However, twelve-step programs don't work for everyone.

There has been little scientific research into the efficacy of cannabis substitution. In his medical cannabis practice, Dr. Mikuriya reported treating 92 alcoholic patients who successfully used marijuana as a substitute [Mikuriya[68]]. However, a clinical investigation by C. M. Rosenberg had disappointing results, concluding that "most alcoholics neither want to substitute marihuana nor find it particularly helpful" [Rosenberg[69]]. Probably just a minority of alcoholics are amenable to marijuana substitution. Furthermore, many users, especially those with addictive tendencies, like to combine marijuana with alcohol and other drugs. Some users even say that pot smoking makes them drink more because it makes them thirsty.

---

68 Mikuriya T, "Cannabis as a Substitute for Alcohol," Journal of Cannabis Therapeutics 3 #1 (2003).
69 Rosenberg CM, et al, "Cannabis in the treatment of alcoholism," J Stud. Alcohol 39:1955-8 (1978).

Still, there is evidence that marijuana may help stem alcohol and other drug abuse. In Jamaica, where ganja (the local term for cannabis) has gained widespread cultural acceptance, investigators found a corresponding decline in heavy alcohol drinking [Rubin[70]]. While the rate of hospital admissions for alcoholism was less than 1% in Jamaica, it was 20%-55% in other neighboring Caribbean islands where ganja was less accepted[71] [Beaubrun]. In the Netherlands, where cannabis is openly sold in coffee shops, the use of illegal drugs is generally lower than in most European countries, leading Dutch health officials to argue that tolerance of cannabis has helped stem hard drug abuse. Studies by the RAND Corporation found that teen marijuana use tends to increase with decreasing access to alcohol, and that states with higher marijuana use have fewer emergency-room visits for drug abuse [Model[72]]. Another study, by Frank Chaloupka of the University of Illinois at Chicago, found that states with liberal marijuana laws tend to have fewer auto accidents than other states, perhaps because they have less drunken driving [Chaloupka[73]].

OTHER APPLICATIONS
Glaucoma

Glaucoma is a disease that causes excess fluid pressure in the eye (IOP–intraocular pressure). Over time, this pressure damages the optic nerve, causing progressive loss of vision and eventual blindness. (Some argue that other factors in addition to increased IOP must be present.) Some patients suffer

70 Rubin V and Comitas L, Ganja in Jamaica pp. 142-6 (Mouton & Co., the Hague,1975).
71 Beaubrun M, "Cannabis or Alcohol: The Jamaican Experience," in Cannabis and Culture, Vera Rubin, Ed., pp. 485-94 (Mouton & Co., the Hague, 1975).
72 Model K, "The Effect of Marijuana Decriminalization on Hospital Emergency Room Episodes," Journal of the American Statistical Association 88.423:737-47 (1993).
73 Chaloupka F & Laixuthal A, "Do Youths Substitute Alcohol and Marijuana? Some Econometric Evidence," National Bureau of Economic Research Working Paper No. 4662, Cambridge, Mass. 1993.

painful, acute attacks with severe headaches and vomiting; in others, visual problems such as halos and blind spots are the most prominent symptoms. Glaucoma is the leading cause of blindness, affecting an estimated two million Americans over 35. It is normally treated by a variety of drugs and surgical procedures, but not always successfully.

It was discovered in the early 1970s that marijuana can help control glaucoma. At the time, it was widely believed that marijuana dilates the pupils of the eyes—a symptom that police hoped would help them uncover marijuana use. A UCLA research team, led by Drs. Robert Hepler and Thomas Ungerleider, tried to find out whether this was so. As part of their tests, they decided to give each subject a complete eye exam. As it turned out, marijuana did not dilate the eyes, but it did cause a significant reduction in IOP [Heppler and Ungerleider[74 75]].

Follow-up studies confirmed that marijuana reduces IOP and can therefore help control glaucoma. Smoked marijuana and intravenously administered THC produced a consistent reduction in IOP of about 20% to 40%, for a period of up to four hours [Adler[76]]. Studies showed that the effects were largely dose-independent, meaning that a heavier dose does not achieve further reduction of IOP. In many, if not all, cases, chronic use doesn't seem to result in tolerance; this implies that marijuana can be used for extended treatment.

Over the years, patients have turned to marijuana for relief from glaucoma when other treatments have failed. Because marijuana is more psychoactive than other glaucoma treatments, it is general-

---

74 Hepler RS and Frank IR, "Marihuana smoking and intraocular pressure," JAMA 217:1392 (1971).

75 Hepler RS, Frank IR, and Ungerleider JT, "Pupillary constriction after marijuana smoking," Am J Ophthalmol. 74:1185-90 (1972).

76 Adler M & Geller E, "Ocular Effects of Cannabinoids," Chapter 3 in R. Mechoulam, ed., Cannabinoids as Therapeutic Agents, CRC Press (1986).

ly used as a last resort. However, numerous patients say they have found relief from marijuana after other treatments have failed.

Among them is Robert Randall, the first patient to obtain legal access to medical marijuana through the FDA. Randall, who had discovered that marijuana alone was able to prevent his sight from deteriorating, launched a lawsuit against the government after losing his home marijuana garden to a police raid. In 1978, he won a settlement in which the government agreed to supply NIDA-grown marijuana free of charge under a special compassionate IND FDA investigational drug protocol. Under the terms of this arrangement, Randall was technically considered to be a research subject in an FDA-approved single-person drug investigation, a process involving elaborate red tape and paperwork for Randall's physician. Difficult as it was for patients to qualify for this program, the compassionate IND protocol was expanded to some 30 patients until it was closed to new applicants by the Bush administration. Today, just four patients still receive marijuana from the government. Though Randall has died, they still include one glaucoma patient, Elvy Musikka.

Despite such well-documented precedents, professional ophthalmologists have resisted endorsing marijuana for glaucoma. In his famous decision recommending that marijuana be rescheduled as a prescription drug, DEA judge Francis Young explicitly excluded glaucoma as an established use for cannabis, citing professional opposition from the American Academy of Ophthalmology, which claimed there was a lack of scientific evidence supporting marijuana's safety and efficacy.

One of the ophthalmologists' major concerns is that glaucoma patients need continual treatment to control their IOP. In Randall's case, this meant smoking some 10 to 12 joints per day. Chain smoking of this kind poses obvious health concerns,

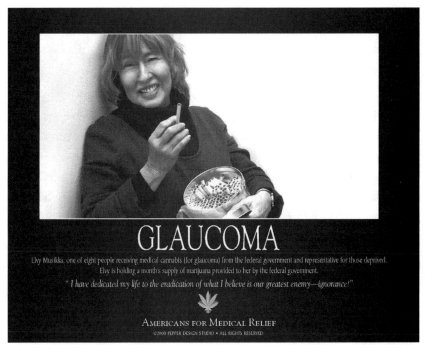

GLAUCOMA

Elvy Musikka, one of eight people receiving medical cannabis (for glaucoma) from the federal government and representative for those deprived. Elvy is holding a month's supply of marijuana provided to her by the federal government.

" I have dedicated my life to the eradication of what I believe is our greatest enemy—ignorance!"

AMERICANS FOR MEDICAL RELIEF
©2000 PEPPER DESIGN STUDIO • ALL RIGHTS RESERVED

This ad by Americans for Medical Relief shows Elvy Musikka, a glaucoma sufferer and one of eight people who receive medical cannabis from the federal government. Elvy holds a month's supply of marijuana provided to her by the government. Elvy, representative for those deprived, says, "I have dedicated my life to the eradication of what I believe is our greatest enemy—ignorance!" *Photo: Larry Utley, © Pepper Design Studio*

especially respiratory hazards, over long periods of time. In addition, patients must spend all of their waking hours under the influence of THC; most subjects find this condition mentally incapacitating. Randall claimed to have developed a tolerance to the psychoactive effects of THC while staying sensitive to its therapeutic effects. Marijuana may be more useful as a nighttime adjunct to standard therapy. Because IOP tends to run higher at night, patients may find it helpful to take a joint just prior to bedtime.

Marijuana is most useful for wide-angle glaucoma, a condition that requires constant treatment. It does not control narrow or closed-angle glaucoma, a condition that manifests itself through acute, painful attacks. Although some patients find that marijuana relieves the pain of these attacks, surgical treatment is essential to preserve vision.

For reasons unknown, glaucoma doesn't respond well to oral THC. Eye patients are virtually unanimous in claiming that Marinol doesn't help them. Surprisingly, laboratory studies have found that pure delta-9-THC does lower eye pressure when administered intravenously. However, a trial of oral THC capsules failed to produce results except at uncomfortably high doses of 20 to 25 mg [Adler[77]]. Animal tests have shown that CBN and delta-8-THC reduce IOP, but CBD does not. This is one of the rare cases in which CBN has proven more medically effective than CBD.

Many patients say that they find low-grade marijuana to be as effective for treating glaucoma as high-potency sinsemilla.

Efforts have been made to develop topical eye drops that would avoid the systemic psychoactive effects of THC. In Jamaica, an eyedropper preparation of cannabis known as Canasol® has been on the market since 1983 for treatment of glaucoma. Due to international restrictions, the drug isn't sold outside Jamaica.

The ocular action of THC is not well understood. THC may reduce pressure by decreasing fluid secretion and/or increasing fluid outflow from the eye. The latter effect may be related to THC's well-known action of dilating the blood vessels in the eyes' conjunctiva. This produces the well-known symptom of bloodshot eyes—a telltale, but unreliable, sign that you've been smoking pot.

Another side effect of THC is to suppress tears. Dry eyes are an annoying problem for some patients. Chronic dryness of the eyes can lead to many other complications, such as cornea ul-

---

77 Adler and Geller, *ibid.*

ceration, conjunctivitis, and keratitis. Some contact lens users say they experience discomfort after smoking marijuana.

Other Ocular Effects

Marijuana is useful for eye diseases other than glaucoma. Edward has used marijuana to treat a drusen cyst, a growth that exerts pressure on his eyeball. Strangely, he says his condition responds to low-grade Mexican grass but not to high-potency sinsemilla. Once again, this indicates that marijuana's medical value depends on more than just THC potency.

Cannabis may also be beneficial for certain eye disorders that are not related to ocular pressure. Some patients say marijuana helps relieve retinitis, an inflammation of the retina. One woman claims that marijuana helps her cope with optic nerve hypoplasia, a congenital underdevelopment of the eye that impairs her vision. She says marijuana helps her focus and see colors better, as well as reducing rapid abnormal eye movements. Other patients have reported that marijuana is useful for vision problems associated with macular degeneration, a progressive deterioration of the retina. Another patient reports that pot has helped him with amblyopic dyslexia, a difficulty with reading caused by blurry vision. As we have seen, CBD may protect against retinal neuropathy or loss of vision caused by diabetes, which may be due to glutamate toxicity.

Several reports suggest that marijuana may improve night vision. Such is the word among Jamaican and Moroccan fisherman, which Dr. Ethan Russo confirmed in a single case study [Russo78]. In another strange example of cannabis-enhanced

---

78 Russo E, "Cannabis improves night vision: a case study of dark adaptometry and scotopic sensitivity in kif smokers of the Rif mountains of northern Morocco," Journal of Ethnopharmacology 93:99–104 (2004).

vision, Dr. Mikuriya reported the case of a color-blind patient whose color vision improved using cannabis.

Asthma

Some patients find marijuana useful for relieving asthma attacks. Asthma is an allergic disorder in which the linings of the lungs become inflamed and swollen with phlegm, causing acute attacks of wheezing and breathlessness. Attacks are treated with bronchodilators, which relax and expand the air passageways of the lungs.

One of the proven effects of THC is to act as a bronchodilator. Studies have found that both smoked marijuana and oral THC can relieve asthmatic spasms. In comparison to standard bronchodilators, marijuana was found to have a milder peak effect, but to act longer. Except for its psychoactivity, marijuana has fewer adverse side effects than other asthma drugs.

An important problem with inhaled marijuana is the smoke. Many asthmatics have a low tolerance for smoking of any kind. The best alternative for asthmatics is therefore probably to vaporize. Another answer is to use oral THC, but the difficulty is its long period of onset. At one point, Dr. Donald Tashkin of UCLA tested a THC spray inhaler for use with asthma. As it turned out, the THC droplets were too irritating when they were inhaled. Other methods of inhaled delivery of pure THC are under development but have not come to market. The closest alternative is GW Pharmaceuticals' Sativex, which isn't inhaled, but sprayed sublingually (under the tongue).

Historically, marijuana was used to treat asthma in Mexican folk medicine. Introduced into the U.S. in the 1910s, this treatment was the first reported medical use of smoked marijuana cigarettes.

A cannabis-based drug known as Asmasol is available in Jamaica for treatment of asthma. The drug is also said to be good for coughs, colds and nausea. Asmasol is not based on THC, but on other components of cannabis. It was developed by Dr. Albert Lockhart and Professor Manley West, who also developed the glaucoma drug Canasol. Like Canasol, Asmasol remains unavailable outside of Jamaica because of international restrictions.

Stroke, Alcoholic Damage, and Brain Injury

As we have seen, cannabinoids have neuroprotective effects against brain and nerve cell damage due to chemical stress and injury. In particular, studies have found that THC and CBD may protect against toxicity from excess glutamate, the excitatory neurotransmitter that is overproduced when cells are damaged. Glutamate toxicity is a cause of cell death in brain injuries and stroke, as well as diseases such as ALS and Alzheimer's. An Israeli pharmaceutical company named Pharmos developed a synthetic CBD analogue known as dexanabinol to treat stroke and brain injuries, but the drug flopped in testing. One problem is delivering the cannabinoids in a timely manner to the endangered cells. There's no reason to think that routine use of inhaled or ingested cannabis can provide substantial protection against stroke or brain damage.

Glutamate toxicity can also be caused by excess alcohol. One study found that CBD protected rats from neurodegeneration due to binge exposure to alcohol [Hamelink[79]]. As we have seen, some alcoholics find that they can alleviate their drinking problem by cannabis substitution. They have good reason to do so, as alcohol is known to kill brain cells, while

---

79 Hamelink C, Hampson A, Wink D, Eiden L, and Eskay R, "Comparison of Cannabidiol, Antioxidants, and Diuretics in Reversing Binge Ethanol-Induced Neurotoxicity," Journal of Pharmacology And Experimental Therapeutics 314:780-788 (2005).

marijuana appears to have the opposite effect.

Possible Anti-Tumoral Effects

There is growing evidence that cannabinoids may have anti-tumoral properties. Experiments with laboratory animals have shown that injections of THC, CBN, and other cannabinoids reduce the size of certain cancers. In particular, studies by Dr. Manuel Guzman at Madrid's Complutense University found that THC inhibited the growth of gliomas, an aggressive form of cancer that attacks the brain and spinal cord, by promoting cell death (apoptosis) and reducing the proliferation of cancerous cells [Guzman[80]]. Similar results were obtained in studies of human glioma cells using CBD. However, these studies involved the direct application of THC and CBD on tumor cells in the lab, not smoking or ingestion of cannabis.

There is growing evidence that various cannabinoids and endocannabinoids can inhibit the proliferation of other cancer cell lines, including, breast, prostate, colorectal, lung and uterine sarcomas, gastric and pancreatic adenocarcinomas, leukemia, and various forms of lymphoma [Armentano[81]]. Many experts believe that cannabinoids may represent a potential new class of anticancer drugs. However, such treatment may require direct application of cannabinoids to the tumor cells, as opposed to inhaling or ingesting marijuana. There is no good reason to assume that use of marijuana normally suppresses cancer in humans. (However, one well-known patient, Steve Kubby, has success-

---

80 Guzman, et al, "A pilot clinical study of delta-9-THC in patients with recurrent glioblastoma multiforme," British Journal of Cancer 95:197-203 (2006); Guzman, et al, "Cannabinoids inhibit the vascular endothelial growth factor pathways in gliomas," Cancer Research 64:5617-23 (2004); Guzman, et al, "Delta-9-THC induces apoptosis in C6 glioma cells," FEBS Letters 436:6-10 (1998).

81 Armentano P, "Emerging Clinical Applications for Cannabis and Cannabinoids: A review of the Recent Scientific Literature 2000-2006," NORML Foundation, Washington DC, Jan 31, 2007. http://www.norml.org

On Medical Marijuana Use

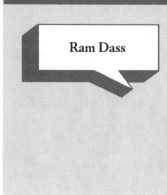

Ram Dass

"First of all, I use medical marijuana for my stroke…to control spastic movements, and for pain. These are my legal reasons for using. But that's the minor use of it. More important, I use marijuana because the stroke captures my consciousness—and I use it to free my consciousness from the stroke. I use it to free my words."

fully used marijuana to control a rare and deadly form of adrenal cancer known as malignant pheochromocytoma.)

Likewise, there is no reason to think that cannabinoids cause cancer. Some anti-pot propagandists alleged this in the 1970s, but such charges have not been born out. An epidemiological survey by Kaiser Health found no higher or lower incidence of cancer in chronic marijuana users [Sidney[82]]. Nonetheless, as we shall discuss later, there remain concerns about the carcinogenicity of certain toxic, non-cannabinoid combustion by-products found in marijuana smoke. These can be avoided by vaporization or oral administration.

---

82 Sidney S, Quesenberry CP Jr, Friedman GD, Tekawa IS, "Marijuana use and cancer incidence (California, United States)," Cancer Causes Control 8:722-8 (1997).

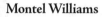

Montel Williams

"When someone suggested I try marijuana, I was skeptical. But I also was desperate. To my amazement, it worked after the legal drugs had failed. Three puffs and within minutes the excruciating pain in my legs subsided. I had my first restful sleep in months.

"You see, people with MS suffer from a particular type of pain called neuropathic pain: pain caused by damage to the nerves. It's common in MS but also in many other illnesses, including diabetes and HIV/AIDS. It's typically a burning or stabbing sensation, and conventional pain drugs don't help much, whatever the specific illness.

"In my case, medical marijuana has allowed me to live a productive, fruitful life despite having multiple sclerosis. Many thousands of others all over this country —less well-known than me but whose stories are just as real—have experienced the same thing.

"Here's what's shocking: The U.S. government knows marijuana works as a medicine. Our government actually provides medical marijuana each month to five patients in a program that started about 25 years ago but was closed to new patients in 1992. One of the patients in that program, Florida stockbroker Irvin Rosenfeld, was a guest on my show two years ago. If federal officials come to town to tell you there's no evidence marijuana is a safe, effective medicine, know this: They're lying, and they know it."

Chapter 4
Adverse Effects, Real and Imaginary

There is so much myth and legend about the dangers of marijuana that it is sometimes difficult for the concerned user to know what to believe. Some people decide that with all the smoke (so to speak) there must be some fire, and they decide against medical marijuana without ever exploring the facts for themselves. At the other extreme, because so many of the alleged dangers are false, some people decide not to believe any of it.

A well-informed middle ground is better. In this chapter we will look into some of the risks commonly ascribed to marijuana and thresh some truth out of them. In broad outline, the claims against marijuana fall into three categories:

+ Situational Concerns: In a few cases the evidence is not clear, or the risks are of real concern to only a few patients.

+ Marijuana Myths: Straight out of Reefer Madness and pot opponents' nightmares, some claims have no rational basis.

+ Real Concerns: It's not all smoke and mirrors. The use of any medication carries some cautions, and marijuana is no exception. When a claim is backed up by genuine medical evidence, the wise user should take that into account.

SITUATIONAL CONCERNS

In some cases the medical evidence is ambiguous. In others there are demonstrable risks but they apply only in specific circumstances. Each patient needs to assess these matters on a case-by-case basis. Here we discuss:

+ Cardiovascular issues associated with marijuana use; marijuana effects on heartbeat and blood pressure

+ Implications for marijuana use during pregnancy and while breast-feeding

+ Possible allergic reactions to marijuana

Cardiovascular Issues

Right after smoking, THC speeds up the heart by as much as 30 to 60 beats per minute. This condition, known as tachycardia, lasts for the first hour or so. There is no reason to think it is dangerous for persons in normal health, any more than the fast heartbeat caused by jogging or by a game of tennis. However, it may be a problem if you have heart disease. Some heart patients experience chest pains or other circulatory discomfort when they smoke marijuana. In this case, of course, they should stop and consult their doctors.

A recent prospective study of patients who had suffered prior heart attacks found an elevated risk of mortality among those who continued to use marijuana, similar to the risk associated with alcohol consumption. The study found a somewhat higher mortality for regular users than occasional users, but the risk applied to deaths due to non-cardiovascular as well as cardiovascular causes, leaving it unclear whether the results were really due to heart stress [Mukamal[1]].

Frequent users may develop tolerance to tachycardia. The prescription drugs known as beta-blockers, which are often prescribed for high blood pressure and other circulatory ailments, can block tachycardia. If you're concerned about tachycardia, you might find it useful to ask your doctor for a beta-blocker prescription if you're thinking of using marijuana.

Tachycardia is likely related to anti-cholinergic effects of marijuana. The cholinergic portion of our nervous system helps regulate heartbeat, body temperature, blood flow and other functions. Many other drugs have anti-cholinergic effects. Tachycardia may be aggravated when THC is combined with certain other drugs, such as nortriptyline, a common antidepressant that also has strong anti-cholinergic effects.

THC may affect blood pressure, but not always in a clear-cut and consistent way. Not uncommonly, THC causes a modest increase in blood pressure for the first few minutes, followed by a modest decrease later. Typically, THC causes a mild increase in blood pressure while lying down and a decrease while standing. However, this doesn't happen for everyone.

Frequently, marijuana causes faintness when one stands up or rises abruptly, a condition known as postural hypotension. Some heavily dosed marijuana users have been known to pass out on the floor. One of the few known stories of a marijuana fatality involved some-

---

1 Mukamal K, et al. "An exploratory prospective study of marijuana use and mortality following acute myocardial infarction," Am Heart J 155(3):465-70 (2008).

one who fell down and cracked his skull on the tub after getting too high. If you feel dizzy or faint, sit or lie down immediately so that you don't fall. Wait for the sensation to pass, then get up gradually.

Studies have suggested that the body's endocannabinoids play a role in modulating blood pressure, with strong doses of cannabinoids having hypotensive (pressure-lowering) effects. However, this hasn't been demonstrated in human clinical studies. The same user may find that THC lowers blood pressure on one occasion, while on another it has the opposite effect. Chronic users may develop tolerance.

For a few patients, THC is clearly helpful in preventing hypertension (high blood pressure). One example is Steve Kubby, a patient advocate from California, who uses marijuana to control a rare, usually fatal form of adrenal cancer. Without THC, Kubby's tumor causes a surge in adrenalin that makes his blood pressure skyrocket. Kubby has been able to prevent this through chronic use of cannabis or Marinol. However, Kubby's condition is unique.

Numerous other hypertensive patients report that they have been able to manage their blood pressure by regular use of marijuana. John reports:

> "Approximately 10 years ago I was diagnosed with high blood pressure. It was so high in fact (155-160 over 95+) it was destroying my one and only kidney. As a kid, I was hyperactive and used to smoke pot to do better in school. It kept me on task. I did a medical trial of my own. A little less than 2 years ago, I started smoking again. My blood pressure has consistently stayed under 130/85, sometimes as low as 120/56. In addition, it has changed my demeanor from anxious and aggressive to caring, gentle, patient, and righteous. In short, the use

of marijuana has saved my kidney, my life my sanity and my family."

Still, surveys of chronic users have not found a statistically significant relation between marijuana use and blood pressure.

In its report, Marijuana and Health (1982), the National Academy of Sciences warned:

> "The smoking of marijuana causes changes in the heart and circulation that are characteristic of stress. But there is no evidence that it exerts a permanently deleterious effect on the normal cerebrovascular system.
>
> "The situation is quite different for a user with an abnormal heart. There is much evidence that marijuana increases the work of the heart. This increase in the workload is dangerous for patients with hypertension, cerebrovascular disease, and coronary atherosclerosis."

The warnings in the NAS report seem remarkably overblown with regards to hypertension, especially in a society where men with cardiovascular disease are commonly prescribed erectile dysfunction medications such as Viagra® or Cialis®, which would seem considerably more risky for the heart. There has never been a reported death from a hypertensive crisis directly attributable to marijuana alone. However, if marijuana is used in combination with more dangerous drugs like cocaine, this can cloud the picture.

Confusingly, the American Glaucoma Society expressed the opposite concern about blood pressure:

"From the standpoint of glaucoma management...the most disturbing adverse reaction is systemic hypotension [low blood pressure], which has been observed with the use of oral and intravenous cannabinoids as well as marijuana inhalation."

Given these conflicting views, the best advice for a heart patient is to talk to your doctor and monitor the effects of marijuana on your own heart rate and blood pressure.

A recent, intriguing animal study suggests that cannabidiol may actually protect the heart [Durst[2]]. As we have seen, CBD is a common non-psychoactive ingredient in marijuana that typically occurs in low concentrations, except in hemp strains and special preparations, such as GW's Sativex spray. CBD appears to have strong anti-inflammatory properties. In the study, rats treated with CBD experienced substantial protection from cardiovascular damage associated with heart attacks.

Pregnancy

In general, women are advised to avoid drugs during pregnancy. This rule applies to marijuana along with all other drugs. However, marijuana isn't so dangerous to fetal health that it can't be used medically when necessary for serious problems such as severe morning sickness.

Marijuana has not been shown to cause gross birth defects. Studies have dispelled concerns, once loudly touted by anti-pot propagandists, that marijuana causes fetal alcohol syndrome and other birth defects. A couple of studies have suggested that marijuana might result in slightly reduced birth weight, which is considered a problem for infant health; however, others have failed to find such an effect. One study even found that marijuana slightly increased birth weight in some instances. A few researchers have suggested that regular maternal marijuana use might slightly retard later development. Here again, though, the

---

2 Durst R et al., "Cannabidiol, a non-psychoactive Cannabis constituent, protects against myocardial ischemic reperfusion injury." Am J Physiol Heart Circ Physiol 293.6:H3602-7 (2007).

evidence is mixed. One study of Jamaican women found improved development scores in children born to ganja-smoking mothers.

In a long-term study, Dr. Peter Fried of Carleton University found that prenatal exposure to cannabis had no effects on young children, but was associated with slightly lower scores on "executive function," or the ability to focus and integrate various mental tasks, when the children reached adolescence. The failure of Dr. Fried's study to find effects at an early age raises questions about its credibility. It has been suggested that cannabinoids could interfere with the way brain cells form new connections. Such effects, if real, are very subtle and have not been confirmed. In any event, Fried concluded that prenatal drug exposure accounts for only 8% of the variance observed in cognitive tests, and this counts alcohol and tobacco along with marijuana. Virtually all studies agree that alcohol and tobacco have worse prenatal effects than marijuana [Morgan[3]].

The therapeutic benefits of medical marijuana must be weighed against these hypothetical risks. Many women find cannabis helpful in relieving morning sickness. In such cases, treatment of severe nausea may be of more importance to fetal health than any slight potential risk from prenatal drug exposure. Obviously, if the mother has a life-threatening disease such as cancer, the risks of fetal exposure to cannabis are of even lesser concern.

Breast Feeding

Some concern has been raised about breast-feeding and marijuana. Since THC is fat-soluble, a small amount makes its way into the mother's breast milk. Studies have found that a fraction of one per cent of a mother's dose of THC might be delivered to

3 For a discussion of Fried's work and prenatal risks of marijuana, see Morgan J & Zimmer L, Marijuana Myths and Marijuana Facts (Lindesmith Center, 1997), pp 103-4.

the baby [Grotenhermen[4]]. One study found no effect of marijuana exposure on infant development; another found slight effects that dissipated after the first month. In any case, the effects would seem negligible except for the very heaviest chronic users.

Allergic Reactions

A few individuals suffer serious adverse effects due to extreme sensitivity or allergic reactions to marijuana. Users have reported such adverse reactions as racing heartbeat, faintness, twitches, numbness, headaches, and rashes. Allergic reactions are not always evident at first, but may require chronic exposure to develop. Workers who trim or handle marijuana regularly have been known to develop skin rashes. If you regularly experience discomforting reactions from marijuana, the best treatment is to avoid it.

MARIJUANA MYTHS

Anti-pot propagandists have attributed many other adverse effects to marijuana (indeed, claims of marijuana's toxicity, once they're made, never die). Many such charges were widely publicized in the 1980s by the government and anti-pot groups, but have since been disproved. Common myths include:

+ Marijuana impairs fertility and reproduction.

+ Marijuana causes brain damage.

+ Marijuana use leads to chromosome and cell damage.

+ Marijuana damages the immune system.

+ Marijuana offers a "gateway" to hard drug abuse.

+ Marijuana use causes violence.

---

4 For further discussion, see Grotenhermen F, "Does THC in breast milk of cannabis using mothers harm the baby?" International Association of Cannabis Medicine. FAQ at: http://www.cannabis-med.org/english/faq/20-breastmilk.htm

Selected Milestones in the History of Pot Hysteria in the U.S.

1901-
1910   First U.S. reports of a menacing new drug from Mexico, "marihuana," allegedly linked to madness and violence. Early reports fail to link it to cannabis indica, a familiar pharmaceutical with a reputation for safety that had been sold in pharmacies since 1850s.

1911   Massachusetts passes the first US law restricting the sale of cannabis. The law outlaws sale of "Indian hemp" except by licensed pharmacists on a doctor's prescription.

1913   Concerned about cannabis-using "Hindoos," California bans Indian hemp. The law is accidentally miswritten so as to outlaw possession of hemp medicines, but is never so enforced.

1914   The first marijuana bust: the California Board of Pharmacy raids Mexican growers in Los Angeles

1915   Utah enforces Mormon religious doctrine by banning marijuana after a band of renegade brethren return from Mexico with the habit.

1919   The first medical marijuana bust: a Mexican maid is arrested in Orange County, CA for growing marijuana to make tea to treat her stomach trouble.

1930   The Federal Bureau of Narcotics is formed, headed by Henry J. Anslinger.

1932   Since 1911, 29 states have criminalized pot. Some laws are based on prejudice against Mexicans, who are viewed as the main users. Others are passed to cut "addicts" off from a drug not restricted by Federal law, like alcohol and narcotics are by that time. The Federal government finalizes the Uniform Narcotic Drug Act, which gives states a standard framework for regulating opiates and cocaine. The Uniform Act makes the production and possession of "narcotic drugs" subject to stringent state licensing. Marijuana is included in the Uniform Act, but only in an optional supplement. All 48 states soon adopt the Uniform Act.

1936   The classic exploitation film *Reefer Madness* premieres.

1937   The Marihuana Tax Act passes the US Congress without a recorded vote. The Tax Act does not explicitly make "marihuana" illegal, but subjects it to a prohibitive tax, rendering it uneconomical even for medical purposes.

1941   The last medical cannabis products disappear from U.S. drugstore shelves.

1948   Actor Robert Mitchum is arrested for possession of marijuana. He serves 60 days behind bars, but is more popular than

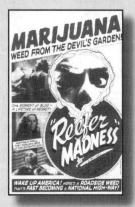

ever when he returns to acting. The conviction is eventually overturned amidst allegations of entrapment.

1951   Congress passes the Boggs Act, which sets harsh mandatory sentences for violations of the Marihuana Tax Act or the Uniform Narcotic Drug Act. State legislatures follow the Federal lead in passing similar laws.

1970   Richard Nixon signs the Controlled Substances Act into law. This massive legislation sets up the modern framework for classifying and regulating both legal and illegal drugs, superseding the Marihuana Tax Act. On the bright side, NORML is founded in this year.

1972   The Presidential Commission on Marihuana and Drug Abuse recommends that marijuana be decriminalized. Nixon ignores it.

1982   Nancy Reagan tells people to "Just Say No."

1988   In September, DEA administrative law judge Francis Young concludes, "marijuana is one of the safest therapeutically active substances known to man." He recommends that marijuana be rescheduled to permit medical use. In November, Ronald Reagan creates the Office of National Drug Control Policy, officially launching the "War on Drugs."

1991   San Francisco voters approve medical marijuana under

Proposition P, by 80% of the vote.

1993   Dennis Peron opens the San Francisco Cannabis Buyers' Club, the first medical cannabis dispensary.

1996   On Nov. 5th, California passes the Compassionate Use Act (Proposition 215) to legalize medical marijuana. Over the next 11 years, 11 more states enact similar measures.

1998   The federal government obtains a court injunction against the Oakland Cannabis Buyers' Club and five other cannabis clubs to block distribution of medical marijuana.

2001   The Supreme Court upholds the injunction against the Oakland Cannabis Buyers' Club. DEA raids the Los Angeles Cannabis Resource Center and a cannabis clinic in El Dorado County, CA. Despite the federal crackdown, dozens of clinics and clubs remain in operation.

2002   The DEA raids Ed Rosenthal, coauthor of this book, and the Wo/Men's Alliance for Medical Marijuana in Santa Cruz for growing medical marijuana.

2003   Rosenthal is sentenced to a single day in jail after the jury recants its guilty verdict on discovering that he was growing for medical purposes. In December, the Ninth Circuit Court of Appeals upholds a lawsuit by two Prop. 215 patients, Angel Raich and Diane Monson, ruling that the federal government cannot arrest medical marijuana patients under its powers to regulate interstate commerce.

2004   Citing the Ninth Circuit's Raich ruling, WAMM wins a federal injunction preventing DEA from raiding its garden – the first legal private cultivation of marijuana in the U.S. since the Marihuana Tax Act.

2005   The Supreme Court strikes down the Ninth Circuit's Raich decision, restoring total prohibition of medical cannabis at the federal level.

1998-   Eleven more states join California in legalizing medical
2007   marijuana

2005-7 Scores of DEA raids on medical marijuana providers fail to prevent over 300 new dispensaries opening up in California and elsewhere.

2007   Ninth Circuit court of Appeals rules Angel Raich has no constitutional right to use marijuana even to save her own life.

Fertility & Reproduction

Experts for the National Institute on Drug Abuse now say that pot has no permanent effect on the male or female reproductive system. Not a single case of impaired fertility has ever been found among marijuana users of either sex. At most, it's possible that marijuana may cause mild, temporary disruptions in ovulation, fertility, and menstrual cycles. Research has also failed to confirm claims that marijuana lowers testosterone and other sex hormones in men or women.

Brain Damage

NIDA experts have also admitted that pot doesn't kill brain cells. This myth was based on some highly questionable animal experiments by Dr. R.G. Heath, in which monkeys were exposed to uncertain levels of smoke. It was disproven by careful research at the National Center for Toxicological Research and SRI International [Morgan[5]]. Human studies in Jamaica and Costa Rica found little evidence of cognitive defects even after long-term, very heavy marijuana use.

Heavy marijuana use does cause measurably lower performance in certain cognitive tasks, such as those involving memory and concentration, verbal fluency, learning ability and recall. These effects can persist for days after last use among heavy users, but eventually subside. Research by Dr. Harrison Pope at McLean Hospital in Belmont, Mass., found cognitive impairment among heavy users at one and seven days after last use, but not after 28 days. Dr. Pope concluded that mental impairment from marijuana is reversible [Pope and Solowij[6]]. Dr. Igor Grant, a professor

---

5 For a discussion on Heath's studies, see Morgan and Zimmer, Marijuana Myths and Marijuana Facts, op. cit., pp. 56-61.
6 Pope H, "Cannabis, Cognition, and Residual Confounding," JAMA 287:1172-1174

of psychiatry at University of California San Diego and director of California's Center for Medicinal Cannabis Research, reaffirmed this conclusion in an analysis of 15 prior studies [Grant[7]]. Dr. Grant was surprised to find that chronic marijuana use did not cause permanent brain damage, given that heavy use of alcohol, amphetamines, and other drugs are known to do so.

Chromosome and Cell Damage

Charges that THC causes chromosome and gene damage are based on outdated studies of the 1970s that have now been conclusively discredited [Morgan & Zimmer[8]].

Immune System

Pot critics have often claimed that THC impairs the immune system. Apparent immunosuppressive effects of THC were first reported in laboratory studies of the 1970s, which found that it mildly inhibited the activity of certain immune cells, in particular T-cells. For the most part, these effects are mild and subtle. Not a single case of human immune system deficiency due to THC has been observed epidemiologically or in clinical studies. As we have seen, studies of HIV and AIDS patients have found no evidence of harmful immunosuppressive effects from marijuana. On the contrary, there is evidence that THC can actually stimulate immune cells and improve T-cell counts.

However, immune suppression may be of concern in certain situations, in particular where the body's immune response is

---

(2002); Solowij N, Stephens RS, Roffman RA, et al, "Cognitive functioning of long-term heavy cannabis users seeking treatment," JAMA 287:1123-1131 (2002).

7 Grant I, et al. "Non-acute (residual) neurocognitive effects of cannabis use: A meta-analytic study," Journal of the International Neuropsychological Society 9.5:679-689 (2003).

8 Morgan and Zimmer, op. cit., p.99.

needed to fight off infections from hostile organisms. To be accurate, cannabinoids do not so much suppress the immune system as modulate it, increasing certain responses and damping others. As explained by Prof. Robert Melamede of the University of Colorado Biology Department, the immune system is balanced between two different pathways known as Th1 and Th2. The Th1 response tends to promote inflammation to fight off infections, while the Th2 response is anti-inflammatory. Cannabinoids tend to suppress the Th1 response and promote the Th2 response. The Th1 response is important for fighting off infectious organisms such as those that cause tuberculosis and Legionnaire's disease. Therefore, it makes sense to avoid marijuana when you need the Th1 system to fight off these and similar infections. On the other hand, marijuana is useful for fighting diseases due to autoimmune inflammation, such as arthritis, rheumatism, diabetes and Crohn's disease, where the Th2 response is helpful.

Some individuals may be particularly susceptible to adverse immune effects. We know of one patient who had genital warts (papilloma virus infection) that resisted treatment whenever he used marijuana. Other lab studies have shown that marijuana may promote herpes infections in animals. On the other hand, some patients insist that marijuana relieves herpes. As always, it's best for patients to be alert for any reactions, both adverse and beneficial.

Unlike oral THC, smoked marijuana impairs the immune response of the lungs. This is not because of the cannabinoids, but because of pyrolytic (combustion-produced) toxins in the smoke, which attack the lung's immune cells, its hair-like cilia, and other defense mechanisms. These hazards can be avoided by taking marijuana orally or by using vaporizers, as described elsewhere in this book.

Gateway to Hard Drug Addiction

One of the most popular myths of anti-pot propagandists is that marijuana use is a "gateway" to hard drug abuse. That is, that using marijuana leads to use of heroin, cocaine, and other addictive drugs. Pharmacologically, there is no basis for this notion. There is nothing about THC that programs the brain to crave harder drugs. The myth derives from the observation that marijuana is often the first illegal drug used by people who go on to use other drugs. Of course, before they try marijuana, most addicts try alcohol or tobacco, not to mention caffeine and mother's milk. The one significant difference is that marijuana is illegal, so that people who obtain it are introduced to criminal dealers, who frequently traffic in other illegal drugs. Thus marijuana is not so much the gateway to addiction as to the illicit drug market.

Scientific investigators have repeatedly rejected the gateway theory. The La Guardia Report was among the first scientific studies to seriously examine the issue [NY Academy of Medicine[9]]. It concluded: "The practice of smoking marihuana does not lead to addiction in the medical sense of the word," and "The use of marihuana does not lead to morphine or heroin or cocaine addiction." More recently, a study of adolescent boys by University of Pittsburgh researchers likewise found that marijuana use is not a reliable predictor of later substance abuse [Tarter[10]].

Harry Anslinger, the notorious head chief of the Federal Bureau of Narcotics, popularized the gateway theory. Ironically, Anslinger initially denied the theory in his testimony to Congress regarding the 1937 Marihuana Tax Act. Asked whether

---

9 Mayor's Committee on Marihuana, the New York Academy of Medicine, "Sociological Study Conclusions" in The LaGuardia Committee Report: The Marihuana Problem in the City of New York–(1944). http://www.druglibrary.org/schaffer/Library/studies/lag/conc1.htm

10 Tarter R, et al: "Predictors of Marijuana Use in Adolescents Before and After Licit Drug Use: Examination of the Gateway Hypothesis," Am J Psychiatry 163:2134-2140 (2006).

there was any connection between marijuana use and addiction to opium or cocaine, Anslinger replied, "No sir: I have not heard of a case of that kind. I think it is an entirely different class. The marijuana addict does not go in that direction" [King[11]]. Later, Anslinger changed his tune. Testifying in favor of the Narcotic Control Act of 1956, which included tougher penalties for marijuana, Anslinger stated, "That is the great problem and our great concern about the use of marijuana, that eventually if used over a long period, it does lead to heroin addiction" [King[12]].

Of course, the fallacy of the gateway theory can be seen in the fact that societies where cannabis is tolerated, such as India, Jamaica, and the Netherlands, have no higher rates of heroin or other hard drug abuse than other countries.

Violence

Contrary to myth, marijuana does not promote violent behavior. If anything, it tends to suppress it. When marijuana first became a public concern in the 1920s, its opponents spread scare stories about reefer-crazed madmen driven to murder and mayhem. These stories were later exposed as fabrications. Instead, subsequent scientific studies found that marijuana tended to promote passivity. This was the finding of New York's LaGuardia Report, which concluded, "There was no aggressiveness or violent behavior observed."

According to the National Academy of Sciences report, "Marihuana and Health," "Both retrospective and experimental studies in human beings have failed to yield evidence that marijuana use leads to increased aggression. Most of these studies suggest quite

---

11 Rufus King, The Drug Hang-Up: America's 50-Year Folly, p.77 (Charles Thomas, Springfield IL, 1974).
12 *Ibid*, p. 90.

the contrary effect. Marijuana appears to have a sedative effect, and it may reduce somewhat the intensity of angry feelings and probability of interpersonal aggressive behavior."

The laid-back hippie, not the murderous bandito, turns out to be the more realistic stereotype of the pot smoker.

REAL CONCERNS

Setting aside all the propaganda, there are still some issues that users should keep in mind when using pot. Conscientious patients can minimize these concerns with a little care. Real issues include:

+ Long-term health effects of marijuana use—primarily damage from smoking and the risk of accidental injury

+ Mental impairment while under the influence

Long-Term Health Concerns

Though marijuana is extremely safe with moderate use, the likelihood of adverse effects naturally rises with long-term, heavy use. Because of the relative novelty of marijuana in developed countries, epidemiological data on its long-term effects are still scarce. Studies of long-term users in Jamaica, Costa Rica, and Greece have found surprisingly little evidence of physiological problems even with extremely heavy use (10 or more joints per day), although they did detect subtle cognitive and psychological defects.

It wasn't till 1993 that a controlled study produced actual epidemiological statistics on the long-term safety of marijuana for users who don't smoke tobacco. The study, conducted by the Kaiser Permanente Center for Health Research, compared the health records of 452 non-tobacco-smoking daily marijuana users with those of 450 non-users [Polen[13]]. It found that the marijuana smokers had a 19% greater risk of respiratory diseases than non-users, confirming the suspicion that marijuana smoking causes lung disease in a way much like that of cigarettes.

The study also found that the daily marijuana smokers had a 30% higher risk of injuries than non-users, suggesting a higher incidence of accidents caused by intoxication. The injury risks were highest for long-term daily marijuana users (15 years or more), but were not significantly higher for newer users.

The authors of the Kaiser study warned that the difficulty of separating the effects of marijuana and alcohol made for complications in their analysis. The subjects who smoked marijuana were much more inclined to be heavy drinkers than the non-users. This was because the heaviest-drinking subgroup of non-users of marijuana, namely tobacco smokers, was excluded. Also, no attempt was made to control for the use of other drugs, such as cocaine, opiates or methamphetamine.

In conclusion, the leading health risks of marijuana appear to be (1) respiratory disease from smoking and (2) accidents resulting from mental impairment. Fortunately, both can be greatly reduced by taking appropriate precautions.

The Act of Smoking

Like tobacco, marijuana smoke is bad for the throat and lungs. Aside from their psychoactive ingredients, marijuana and tobacco smoke are chemically similar; both contain toxins that are known to be hazardous to the respiratory system. These chemi-

---

13 Polen M, et al. (Kaiser study): "Health Care Use by Frequent Marijuana Smokers Who Do Not Smoke Tobacco," West J Med 1993:158.

cals have nothing to do with THC or other cannabinoids; they are non-psychoactive byproducts of leaf combustion. Among them are the carcinogenic compounds known as polycyclic aromatic hydrocarbons (PAHs), which are thought to be a major factor in smoking-related cancers. Marijuana tars are somewhat higher in PAHs than tobacco on a weight-for-weight basis, and have been shown to be carcinogenic in laboratory cell culture studies. In addition, pre-cancerous cell changes have been observed in the respiratory tracts of long-term, heavy marijuana smokers. Despite this, studies on marijuana smoking and cancer have so far come up with less than damning results. Studies of this kind are generally complicated by the fact that many marijuana smokers have also smoked tobacco, making it difficult to separate the effects of marijuana and tobacco. However, as we shall see, the largest studies to date have failed to find a relation between marijuana-only smoking and cancer.

Unlike tobacco, there is little evidence linking marijuana to non-respiratory forms of cancer such as bladder, colon, and rectal cancers. As we shall see, this may be due to chemical differences in tobacco and marijuana smoke, as well as the generally lower smoke consumption of marijuana users.

In addition to the solid tars, marijuana smoke includes gaseous toxins that are thought to be risk factors in heart and respiratory disease. Among these are hydrogen cyanide, carbon monoxide, nitrogen oxides, phenols, and volatile aldehydes.

Human studies have shown that heavy marijuana users have a higher risk of respiratory disease, including bronchitis, sore throat, and other infections. Oddly, the Kaiser study found that these risks were highest in users who had been using marijuana for less than 10 years, whereas longer-term users showed no greater risks than non-smokers. The authors suggested a possible explanation: users with respiratory problems may be more likely to quit early.

The Kaiser study was not large enough to detect smoking-related cancer. Data on marijuana use and cancer are still not entirely definitive because marijuana only came into popularity in recent decades, and so there are still relatively few long-term, elderly users. In the early 1990s, certain specialists began reporting a higher than expected incidence of throat, neck and oral cancers in younger, marijuana-only smokers. Dr. Paul Donald of the University of California at Davis observed that marijuana use seemed even more prevalent than tobacco smoking among his throat cancer patients who were under age 40 [Donald[14]]. However, other researchers disputed the link between marijuana and throat and oral cancers. A more recent study of 407 patients by researchers at the Fred Hutchinson Cancer Research Center found no relation between marijuana smoking and oral cancers. However, study author Karin Rosenblatt cautioned, "Our study isn't the last word on whether there are certain genetic factors that may put people who smoke marijuana at an increased risk of cancer" [Rosenblatt[15]].

Though less deadly than lung cancer, throat and oral cancers can be fatal or disfiguring. Whatever the role of marijuana, tobacco smoking and heavy alcohol drinking are known to aggravate the risk of throat and oral cancers. Patients are therefore well advised to avoid heavy drinking and tobacco smoking.

Recent scientific studies show that marijuana smoking is a lesser hazard to the lungs than tobacco. For many years, it was widely as-

---

14 Donald P, "Advanced malignancy in the young marijuana smoker," Adv Exp Med Biol 288:33-56 (1991); Taylor FM, "Marijuana as a potential respiratory tract carcinogen," South Med Journal 81:1213-6 (1988).
15 Fred Hutchinson Cancer Research Center press release, Jun 1, 2004. For the study itself, see Rosenblatt, K et al, "Marijuana Use and Risk of Oral Squamous Cell Carcinoma." Cancer Research 64:4049-54 (2004).

sumed that marijuana posed similar or worse lung cancer risks than tobacco. This assumption was upset by the first large-scale epidemiological study of marijuana smoking and lung cancer in 2005 by a team of researchers led by Dr. Mia Hashibe and Dr. Paul Tashkin at the University of California at Los Angeles [Hashibe[16]]. In a survey of 1,209 patients with lung, oral, laryngeal and esophageal cancers, the team found no relation between marijuana smoking and cancer. Dr. Tashkin, a leading expert on smoking-related disease, fully expected to find a high cancer incidence from marijuana smoking. Much to his surprise, he found no increased cancer risk even in heavy long-term users. In at least one category–lung cancer among relatively short-term users - the data even showed lower cancer rates for marijuana smokers than non-users.

In another study, Harvard researchers found that THC inhibited the growth and spread of lung cancer tumors in laboratory mice [Preet[17]]. Researchers found that THC blocks a molecule known as epidermal growth factor, which especially promotes the growth of aggressive small-cell lung cancers. The study suggests that THC and other cannabinoids should be explored as possible therapies for suppressing growth and metastasis of certain cancers.

This isn't necessarily the end of the story. Researchers in New Zealand recently reported evidence of heightened lung cancer risk among chronic pot smokers in a case-control study of 79 young patients [Aldington[18]]. As often happens, the study was wildly misreported in the press to imply that pot smoking is more

---

16 Hashibe M, Morgenstern H, Cui Y, Tashkin DP, Zhang ZF, Cozen W, Mack T, and Greenland S, "Marijuana Use and the Risk of Lung and Upper Aerodigestive Tract Cancers: Results of a Population-Based Case-Control Study," Cancer Epidemiol Biomarkers Prev 15.10:1829–34 (2006).

17 Preet A, Ganju RK, Groopman JE, "Delta-9)-Tetrahydrocannabinol inhibits epithelial growth factor-induced lung cancer cell migration in vitro as well as its growth and metastasis in vivo," Oncogene 27:339–346 (2008).

18 Aldington S, et al, "Cannabis use and risk of lung cancer: a case-control study," Eur Respir J 31:280-286 (2008).

dangerous than cigarettes and could cause a cancer epidemic. In fact, the study found practically no difference in lung cancer risk among the pot-smoking subjects. Occasional and moderate marijuana smokers actually showed reduced lung cancer risk. Only those who had smoked daily for ten years or more showed an elevated risk, though less than that for tobacco smokers. All but 9 of the 79 subjects had also smoked tobacco, a population too small to draw definitive conclusions about marijuana-only smoking. Nonetheless, the researchers concluded, "the results of the present study indicate that long-term cannabis use increases the risk of lung cancer in young adults."

As of this date, the risks of respiratory cancers due to marijuana smoking remain uncertain, though the balance of evidence shows they are less than had been expected. Nevertheless, whatever its carcinogenic hazard, marijuana smoke clearly aggravates the risk of other respiratory diseases, including bronchitis, infections, sore throat, etc. In addition, many non-users object to the smell and presence of second-hand smoke. For all of these reasons, heavy users are well advised to seek alternative delivery forms, such as vaporization or edibles.

Marijuana Versus Tobacco

One popular myth spread by "pothibitionists" is that one or two joints per day are equivalent to a pack-a-day cigarette habit. In truth, according to Dr. Tashkin's research, daily marijuana smokers show less evidence of respiratory damage than pack-a-day cigarette smokers. Furthermore, unlike tobacco, there is no evidence linking marijuana to heart disease or to non-respiratory cancers such as bladder, colon, and rectal cancer.

Why should marijuana smoking be less physically harmful than cigarette smoking? One obvious reason is that marijuana smokers consume much less smoke. A typical marijuana user smokes one or two joints a day, whereas a typical tobacco smoker consumes a pack or two of 20 cigarettes per day.

In practice, this must be adjusted for the fact that marijuana smokers tend to inhale more deeply, exposing them to a greater quantity of smoke per puff. A study by Drs. Tashkin and T.-C. Wu found that marijuana smokers absorb between three and five times as much smoke toxins as tobacco smokers per weight smoked [Tashkin[19]]. Therefore, one gram of marijuana is equal to three to five grams of tobacco. In practice, marijuana joints vary greatly in weight, from cigar-sized leaf "blunts" to slender sinsemilla joints weighing a fraction of a gram. In general, the higher quality of the marijuana, the smaller the size of the joint. Using reasonably good quality marijuana, the typical joint weighs 0.4 grams, about half as much as a cigarette. At this rate, the average joint is equivalent to between 1.5 and 2.5 cigarettes.

A second difference between marijuana and tobacco is that tobacco smoke tends to penetrate more deeply into the lungs. For whatever reason, marijuana smoke particles tend to concentrate in the larger, upper air passageways of the lungs and throat, while tobacco penetrates to the smaller, lower passageways. According to Dr. Tashkin, one result of this is that marijuana by itself doesn't appear to cause emphysema, a progressive, degenerative disease of the lower lungs that is linked to tobacco smoking. On the other hand, the combination of marijuana plus tobacco may aggravate the risk of emphysema [Tashkin[20]]. Marijuana may also be more apt to irritate the throat than cigarettes.

---

19 Wu T-C, Tashkin D. et al, "Pulmonary Hazards of Smoking Marijuana as Compared to Tobacco," New England Journal of Medicine 388:347-51 (1988).
20 Tashkin D, et al, "Heavy Habitual Marijuana Smoking Does Not Cause an Accelerated Decline in FEV1 With Age," Am J Respir Crit Care Med 155:141-8 (1997).

A final, major difference between marijuana and tobacco smoke is their principal active ingredients. Marijuana contains THC and other cannabinoids, while tobacco contains nicotine. As we have seen, there is evidence that THC and cannabinoids have cancer-suppressive qualities. On the other hand, nicotine has properties that tend to promote cancer. In addition, other nicotine derivatives in tobacco smoke, such as NNK and NNN, are known to be potent carcinogens. Finally, nicotine is a powerful, addictive vasoconstrictor and stimulant that is known to promote circulatory and heart disease.

According to Prof. Melamede, there are biochemical reasons why cannabis smoke is not as carcinogenic as tobacco [Melamede[21]]. First, THC acts to suppress the conversion of polycyclic aromatic hydrocarbons in marijuana smoke into active carcinogens, whereas nicotine has the opposite effect. Second, nicotine tends to inhibit the destruction of diseased cells (apoptosis), while cannabinoids don't. Third, nicotine promotes the growth of blood vessels feeding tumors (angiogenesis), while cannabinoids tend to have the opposite effect. Dr. Melamede concludes, "It is possible that as the cannabis-consuming population ages, the long-term consequences of smoking cannabis may become more similar to what is observed with tobacco. However, current knowledge does not suggest that cannabis smoke will have a carcinogenic potential comparable to that resulting from exposure to tobacco smoke."

Accidents

The single greatest health concern for most marijuana users is the risk of accidents caused by impairment. Marijuana has ad-

---

21 Melamede R, "Cannabis and tobacco smoke are not equally carcinogenic." Harm Reduction Journal 2:21 (18 Oct 2005).

verse effects on mental concentration and psychomotor skills that are related to driving and other activities. Although the dangers of marijuana are less than those of drunken driving, they're still real. Contrary to the myth that no one has ever been hurt by using marijuana, there's no doubt that some accident fatalities have occurred. Accidents result from careless and irresponsible use and can be avoided given a proper appreciation for marijuana's effects.

Driving simulator studies have consistently found that marijuana adversely affects certain driving skills, in particular tracking ability, or the ability to maintain a constant speed and distance from other cars; attentiveness; judgment of speed and distance; peripheral vision; and coordination at complex tasks. Balance and muscle steadiness are also adversely affected.

Marijuana doesn't noticeably interfere with simple coordination or reaction time—for instance, the ability to put on the brakes quickly. However, it does impair coordination and slow reaction time at complex tasks when prompt decision making is needed—for instance, choosing whether to swerve right or left to avoid an obstacle, or whether to speed up or stop at a crossing when a speeding train is approaching. In general, marijuana is not as dangerous in routine driving as in emergency situations.

Off the road, the greatest danger of marijuana is its adverse effect on concentration and short-term memory. Users may forget important safety procedures, leave the water running or the stove turned on, lose their keys, and so on. Marijuana is to be avoided while doing jobs that require concentration, such as airline traffic control or operating complex machinery. In some instances, heavy chronic users may develop a degree of tolerance to these effects. However, an impaired user is not the best judge of his own impairment. It is best to err on the side of caution.

One of the most disconcerting effects of marijuana is that it makes familiar things seem strange. Drivers may suddenly find themselves lost in familiar neighborhoods or forget to take the right freeway exit.

Fortunately, marijuana users are usually quite aware of their condition and try to compensate for it. Many drivers tend to slow down under the influence of marijuana. In fact, many police consider slow driving to be a telltale sign of marijuana use. In this respect, marijuana differs significantly from alcohol, which tends to provoke speeding and reckless behavior.

In a study of marijuana and driving, National Highway Transportation Safety Administration (NHTSA) researchers concluded that marijuana produces a modest, dose-related reduction in road tracking performance, whose effects are "in no way unusual compared to many medicinal drugs." It found that even at higher doses, marijuana had smaller adverse effects on driving than alcohol at .08% blood alcohol content. The legal threshold for driving under the influence of alcohol typically ranges from .08% to .10%.

Numerous other accident studies have confirmed that marijuana is a lesser driving danger than alcohol. A comprehensive survey of 10 years of U.S. accident data found that alcohol-free drivers with marijuana in their system had a "slightly elevated" risk of unsafe driving behavior, but lower than that for drivers with legal amounts of alcohol in their blood [Bédard[22]]. Similar results were reported in a large-scale study in France [Laumon[23]].

Other studies have found that marijuana is significantly more hazardous in the first hour or two of acute intoxication, when higher

---

22 Bédard M, et al, "The impact of cannabis on driving," Canadian Journal of Public Health 98.1:6-11 (2007).
23 Laumon B, et al, "Cannabis intoxication and fatal road crashes in France: a population base case-control study," British Medical Journal 331:1371-1377 (2005).

concentrations of THC are found in the blood [Drummer[24], Grotenhermen[25]].

In a 1992 National Highway and Transportation Safety Administration study of 1,882 fatal driving accidents, alcohol was found in the blood of 51.5% of all victims, versus 6.7% for marijuana [NHTSA[26]]. Two thirds of the marijuana-using drivers also had alcohol in their systems. After analyzing the accidents in which marijuana alone was involved, NHTSA concluded that "there was no indication that marijuana by itself was a cause of fatal accidents."

On the other hand, the combination of alcohol and marijuana was definitely dangerous. Most driving studies agree that the adverse effects of marijuana and other drugs are additive. In a California survey of young males killed in driving accidents, 80% of marijuana-related fatalities also involved alcohol [Williams[27]]. Evidently, marijuana users are well advised to avoid alcohol and other drugs on the road.

Marijuana causes significant psychomotor impairment for the first couple of hours after smoking. After that, the effects fade. A few studies have detected subtle effects for four to eight hours, but these don't seem to be a major safety concern. One research team claimed to find very subtle effects of marijuana for up to 24 hours on airline flight simulator tests, but other studies have not confirmed these effects [Yesavage[28]].

If you've used marijuana recently, you may want to check yourself

---

24 Drummer OH, et al, "The involvement of drugs in drivers of motor vehicles killed in Australian road traffic crashes," Accident Analysis and Prevention 36:239-248 (2004).
25 Grotenhermen et al. "Developing science-based per se limits for driving under the influence of cannabis." http://www.canorml.org/healthfacts/DUICreport.2005.pdf (2005).
26 US Department of Transportation, National Highway Traffic Safety Administration. The Incidence and Role of Drugs in Fatally Injured Drivers: Final Report. October 1992.
27 Williams A, Peat M, Crouch D, Wells JK, Finkle B, "Drugs in Fatally Injured Young Male Drivers," Public Health Reports 100:19-25 (1985).
28 Yesavage JA, et al, "Carryover effects of marijuana intoxication on aircraft pilot performance: A preliminary report," American Journal Of Psychiatry 142:1325-9 (1985).

Motivation

Marijuana has been said to cause an "amotivational syndrome," characterized by a loss of ambition, motivation, and interest. The evidence for this is disputed. Believers cite examples of adolescents who have suddenly lost interest in school, friends, and so on after starting to smoke pot. Skeptics counter that marijuana doesn't induce amotivation, but that persons who already have motivational problems may be °attracted to heavy marijuana use. They note that many highly motivated and successful professionals are pot smokers.

Marijuana has sedative, relaxing properties. Animal studies have shown that monkeys are less likely to strain for a banana after being given marijuana. (Of course, the monkeys may realize there's no point in knocking themselves out for a lab experiment!) This may explain the "laid-back" stereotype of human potheads. However, it doesn't show that marijuana robs adults of their careers, families, or goals. If you already have a clear sense of goals, using marijuana for medicine won't "demotivate" you. On the other hand, for young adolescents, chronic use can become an escape mechanism that detracts from the pursuit of more worthwhile goals.

before driving. If you find yourself losing track of conversations or forgetting what you were about to say, you're too stoned to drive well. One simple test for motor coordination is to try to talk while standing on one foot. If you lose your balance, you're probably stoned. Another test is to extend your arms to both sides and close your eyes, then draw in each hand and try to touch your nose with your fingertip. If you miss, you're too stoned to drive.

Intoxication and Mental Impairment

For most users, the most important adverse effect of marijuana is mental impairment due to intoxication.

Marijuana seriously interferes with such mental skills as memorization, recall, attentiveness, tracking ability, and coordination at complex tasks. Many users have trouble trying to work, study, or perform difficult tasks while under its influence. Some users develop a tolerance to these effects after a period of chronic use, or learn to compensate and adjust their performance satisfactorily. Some folks manage to go about their everyday lives, more or less satisfactorily, under the continual influence of cannabis. Of course, some of them may be impaired in certain ways without knowing it.

Some people claim that marijuana actually improves their performance, especially at tasks requiring creativity, personal interaction, or rote, repetitive work where boredom is a problem. Scientific studies have failed to support these claims. Still, it is interesting that at one time mine and plantation owners in South America and Africa encouraged workers to take a cannabis break to boost morale and productivity!

Marijuana use has no detectable effect on normal intellectual performance when you're not under the influence. Some people have claimed that heavy use is linked to a decline in so-called "executive functioning," the ability to concentrate and focus your efforts on particular goals. Psychological tests generally do show that heavy pot users are more easily distracted and less attentive to maintaining a course of action.

In any case, problems of this kind are a matter of recreational abuse and aren't generally relevant to medical users. Many patients find marijuana essential to their daily functioning, relieving them from the distractions of pain, discomfort, and debilitating suffering.

Chapter 5
Growing Medicinal Marijuana

You would think that once a state recognized marijuana as a medicine it would develop a system to make it easy for patients to obtain it. That hasn't happened. California is presently the only state that officially allows dispensaries to sell the herb (in some locales). Patients elsewhere must produce their own medicine, have a caretaker do it for them, or purchase it from the black market.

Deciding whether or not a patient should cultivate marijuana or have a caregiver grow it for them requires serious thought, and the grower candidate must consider many factors.

Is there the space to grow? A garden usually takes a minimum of about 9 square feet (0.8 square meter), which is a space 3 feet x 3 feet (0.9 x 0.9 meter). Outdoors a single plant uses anywhere from 4-25 square feet (0.4 to 2.3 square meters).

Does the patient or the caregiver feel confident about his/her horticultural abilities? Although marijuana is not hard to grow, it can be extremely stressful to embark on a project when you are dubious about its outcome.

Does the patient use enough medicine to make cultivation worthwhile? If the patient uses very small amounts of marijuana, it may not make sense either in terms of effort or economically. For instance, if the patient uses only a quarter ounce a month, the time and effort of setting up a garden and maintaining it may not make sense, since the time, effort, and risk may be worth $1,000 a year or so to many people.

Does the patient feel uncomfortable about growing such a controversial plant? In some states cultivation is legal with a doctor's recommendation. Even there, patients run a risk of arrest if their gardens attract adverse attention from the neighbors, unfriendly relatives and acquaintances, landlords, or the cops. If patients feel uncomfortable about possessing a plant that some members of society frown upon, perhaps they should not have a marijuana garden.

Potential growers must face the reality or paranoia of knowing that even where it is legal, the authorities do not look benevolently upon medical marijuana, and innocent patients have been arrested or hassled for its use.

Gardener candidates should also be aware that marijuana is a very seductive plant. It completes its lifecycle, from seed or cutting to ripeness and senescence in a quarter year or less. Each day of a marijuana plant's life is the equivalent of a year in human terms. Marijuana is also dioecious, meaning that male and female flowers grow on separate plants and (unlike most birds and mammals but like humans) the female form is sought for its beauty. It is not uncommon for gardeners to become obsessed with growing this plant. From my observations of marijuana growers, I have come to the conclusion that using marijuana is not addictive, but growing it is.

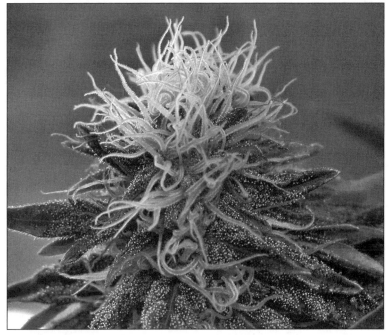

Mid-stage flower. *Photo: Seemorebuds*

Aside from the legal paranoia, growing marijuana is a very rewarding and pleasant experience. It is fast growing and responds very quickly to changes in environmental conditions. Over a season you will experience the complete life of a living organism that has lived symbiotically with humans for so long that scientists don't think that wild marijuana exists.

Feral marijuana (hemp) is found in the Himalayas and across the Caucasus as well as in the U.S. Midwest. Even though it is weedy and grows without human aid, sometime in the past its progenitors intersected with humans, which caused permanent changes in its evolution. The symbiotic relationship has had a profound effect on both species.

For cannabis, the evolving relationship helped it spread from its home in the Himalayan valleys to every continent on the planet. For humans, cannabis provided shelter, clothing, food, medicine and change of consciousness.

Not content with growing the plant outdoors, in the past half-century humans have bred varieties that thrive indoors under artificial lighting. Today, in the California dispensaries, indoor grown marijuana is priced higher than outdoor because of the higher quality and consistency of the indoor buds.

THE PLANT

Marijuana is a sun-loving/light-loving annual plant that thrives in rich, well-drained soil such as well-prepared garden soil. It is a heavy feeder and does best in moist rather than dry mediums. Varieties have been bred to thrive under many conditions so that gardeners indoors and out, in small spaces and large, have appropriate varieties to choose from.

Many people picture marijuana in their mind's eye as a giant plant that spreads out eight or ten feet in diameter and towers above the people standing next to it. Outdoor gardeners sometimes grow large plants like these; however, marijuana comes in many sizes and shapes and is often harvested ripe at two to three feet in height. There are thousands of varieties, and they vary in size, shape, color, potency, and their favored environmental conditions. They also vary in their medicinal properties.

When gardeners in the U.S. first started growing marijuana, they relied on varieties from Central and South America, Southeast Asia, the Himalayas and Africa. These landlines have been bred and adapted by home gardeners and commercial breeders. Today's marijuana grows faster and ripens earlier, produces more and is easier to grow than varieties from only a few years ago. There are more choices of medicinal qualities and they are often more potent than the older varieties, which required considerable huffing and puffing to provide medical relief.

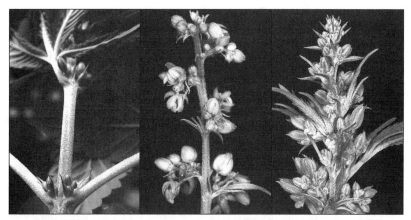

Male plants *Photos: Ed Rosenthal*

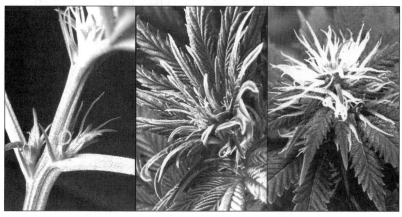

Female plants *Photos: Ed Rosenthal, Seemorebuds (middle photo)*

Life Cycle

Marijuana germinates in the spring. Given sun, warmth, rich soil, fertilizers and adequate water, and left untrimmed, it will quickly grow into one of its typical forms, which include: bushy, Christmas tree shaped, or much like a fir tree-shaped, with short branches around a central stem, or tall with little branching.

It continues to grow leaves until August, when the days grow shorter and the nights longer. The plant measures the length of the uninterrupted dark period each evening. When the dark period reaches a critical length the plant redirects its energy from stem and leaf growth to flowering. The male plants produce flowers just as the females are becoming receptive.

Males produce small, five-petal, white or yellow flowers on long spikes and along some of the branches. Before they open the immature flowers look something like pawnbroker balls, hanging down from their stems. As they open the flowers change position to upright, so the petals face the skyward. The mature pollen catches the wind and drifts off to pollinate the female flowers. After flowering, male plants lose vigor and die.

Since it is wind-pollinated, there is no reason for the female to produce a fancy flower with petals. Instead, each flower produces two stigmas that stick out into the air. Thousands of flowers grow all along the branches. Eventually leafy areas are filled with tightly packed layers of flowers. When a pollen grain floats by it sticks to a stigma. The pollen's DNA sac quickly passes down a hollow tube in the stigma to the ovum found in the ovary, behind the flower. Fertilization is complete and the seed begins to grow. When most of the flowers have been pollinated the plant slows growth of flowers and switches its energy to producing viable seeds. They mature in about three weeks and eventually fall to the ground as the seed pods dry. The plants then lose vigor but hang on until they are killed by frost.

Humans altered this natural process, which served the plants well for tens or hundreds of thousands of years, in order to produce sinsemilla buds. The term comes from two Spanish words- sin, which means without, and semilla, which means seed. Male and female flowers are found on separate plants. This characteristic is unique to cannabis among annual plants.

Sinsemilla buds are prized because of their high potency and

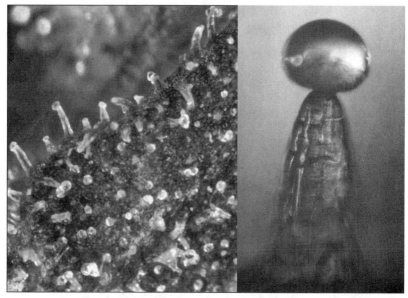

Close-up of trichomes *Photos: Ed Rosenthal*

smooth pleasant smoking qualities. They are the coveted part of the cannabis plant.

When male plants are removed as soon as they indicate sex but before the flowers mature, the flowers on the female plants remain unpollinated. Instead of putting their energy into seed production, the female plants continue to grow more flowers. The budded branches, called colas, sometimes become so thick with flowers that they need support to prevent them falling from the plant. These flowers, all bunched together, are rich in resins that contain THC, the main active component of marijuana.

The groups of flowers growing on the colas are called buds. After growing for five or six weeks the buds' ripening begins. First the stigmas dry and turn color as new flower growth slows to a small fraction of its peak. The stigmas usually turn a saturated orange red, but can also be touched with purple, pink or yellow tones. Then the ovaries behind the stigmas begin to swell as if they were producing seeds. At the same time the glands take on a significant roll.

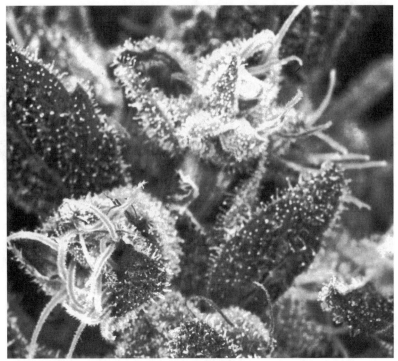

Resinous trichomes on a maturing bud *Photos Ed Rosenthal*

Shortly after germination the plants start producing tiny glands (15-30 microns in diameter) along the stems and on the leaves. These glands, called bulbous trichomes, have a very short stem and a small head, and this is where where THC—the main psychoactive ingredient in marijuana—is manufactured and stored. THC has no odor. The odors are caused by terpenes, which are also manufactured and stored in these glands. When plants are young, these glands are very small and the plants have just a faint odor.

THC and the terpenes are used by the plants for protection from insects, other herbivores and from bacterial and fungal attacks. They may also protect the plants from fungal and bacterial attacks. One of the ways that THC might protect the plant is by locking onto anandamide receptors of herbivore mammals and lizards. Most animals find the sensations unpleasant and learn to avoid the plant, but unfortunately deer appreciate young, pre-flowering marijuana plants.

Immature plants also produce a larger gland that contains the same cannabinoids and terpenes as the bulbous glands. Capitate-sessile glands have a short stalk with a big head attached so they appear to lie on the leaf surface. They are two to three times as large as the bulbous glands.

Both of these glands protect the leaves and stem from predation. However, as the plant starts to grow flowers it has already invested energy into vegetative growth, which is now irreplaceable. It is entering the most crucial stage, reproduction. This investment it has already made and the possibility of seed production are worth protecting with more deterrent.

The plant produces a third kind of trichome, the capitate stalked gland, which appears early in flowering but becomes more prevalent as the flowers grow and mature. These glands stand upright on a stem 200-400 microns long. As the flowers mature the heads of the glands, which consists of a membrane holding THC and plant oils, stretches and looks like a balloon about to burst.

As the flowers mature the liquid in the glands begins to turn cloudy or opaque. The enlarged ovary with the glands covering becomes luminescent in the light. At this point the bud is ready to cut.

Acquiring Seeds and Clones

If you have the occasional stray seed from a sinsemilla bud there is a good chance that it will contain genes for hermaphroditism. That is, the same plant has both male and female flowers. The problem is that the male flowers' pollen will pollinate the females and flower growth will slow down or cease as the plant puts its energy into seed production. That may be how the seed got into the bud in the first place.

The other possibility is that the flower was pollinated by stray pollen. You may have an idea of the mother's background, but there is no telling about the male. Nevertheless, you would assume that both the plants are high quality. After all, why would someone grow a low quality plant? On the other hand you may have little idea of the plant's environmental preferences.

Seed from Mexican marijuana is usually not a good candidate for cultivation. The varieties grown there are much lower quality, that is, they are much less potent because they contain less THC than domestic marijuana. Whether you grow a mediocre variety or a high quality hybrid you use the same equipment, energy and effort. At harvest, your efforts are more amply rewarded when you start with the high quality variety.

Once you have sampled different varieties and have selected the ones that are most efficacious medically, it is time to acquire the genetics. Rather than settling for a strain that is not good medicine for you, try to obtain the ones that you want.

There are two ways to start your garden: seeds and clones. Seeds have the advantage of being easily transportable and shippable. They are widely available through the Internet. To find them look under "marijuana seeds." Several services such as *rollitup.org, weedbay.net* and *weedtracker.com* rate the seed companies and the reliability of their distributors. Seeds are not legal in the U.S. so the companies are located in Canada and Europe.

Seeds result from the combination of genes from separate male and female flowers. So they are not exact genetic duplicates of the mother plant. The plants that are grown from them will not be as homogeneous as a commercial pack of flower or vegetable seeds. As gardeners grow the plants and then again after they sample the harvest, they pick the best plants to continue by taking cuttings and rooting them. They keep only the clones of the selected plants.

Unlike any other annual plant cannabis is dioecious; it has separate male and female plants. Only the female plants are productive, so the males are eliminated. This is tedious and if not done correctly can produce undesirable seeded buds. Some breeders offer "feminized" seed. They are created using techniques that induce female plants to produce pollen. With these seeds gardeners don't have to worry about eliminating males.

Clones are rooted cuttings taken from selected female plants. They have the same genetics as the plant from which they were taken. The advantage of this is that you know that the plant is female and it gets you past the germination hump, just as many gardeners prefer to start with young plants rather than germinate seeds.

If you have the chance to start with clones from a variety you have chosen, that is the better choice. Most professional cloners take their work seriously and choose the best plants and continually upgrade their selections.

Unfortunately, clones and cuttings are not usually available by mail order. However, if you live in California or another state that permits patient cooperatives, or if you know someone who is already growing a variety that you find helpful, you may have access to clones.

There are many seed companies that ship from either Canada or Europe to the United States. These transactions are illegal for both the buyer and the seller. However, the items being smuggled in are so small and so discreetly packaged that it is very rare that the packages are detected. Several magazines, such as *Cannabis Culture*, *High Times* and *Skunk*, feature advertisements from seed companies. A small number of patients' co-ops and dispensaries in medical marijuana states supply domestically produced seeds.

GROWING YOUR OWN MEDICINE
Starting From Seeds or Clones

If you are starting with seeds, they should be germinated indoors four to eight weeks before they are placed outdoors. Start them using high quality store-bought pasteurized planting mix in four-inch plastic containers. Alternatives are Oasis® rooting cubes, Jiffy® pellets, or rockwool cubes. All work well. Place the seeds about ⅛ to ¼ inch into the medium and keep the soil moist. Place the containers under bright compact fluorescents (CFL) with one 60-watt equivalency CFL per square foot. Keep the light on about 18 hours a day if you are planting outdoors and continuously if the plants will be kept indoors. The seeds germinate in three to seven days. Once germination has taken place, continue to keep the soil moist, not wet, and use houseplant fertilizer as recommended.

If you have not started with seeds that are manipulated to produce only females, about half the plants will be males, which will be discarded as soon as they are discovered. It's easier to sex the plants before they are transplanted.

To hasten sex determination, wait until the clones have developed several branches. Remove a side branch from each plant and mark both cutting and plant so they can be matched. Place the cuttings in moist planting mix, Oasis® cubes, or a jar of water filled with one inch of water (replace the water every two or three days). Place the cutting in a moderately lit area and give them only eight hours of light daily on a regular basis. In 10 to 15 days all the cuttings will grow either male or female flowers. Match the cuttings to the plants, identify the males and discard them.

If you are starting with clones from a dispensary or grower, you know that all the plantlets are female and have hopefully been selected for the high quality buds they produce. They can be transplanted as soon as they are well rooted.

Growing Outdoors

You can plant marijuana outdoors in the late spring through the middle of July. The earlier you plant, the bigger the plant will grow. Starting plants late outdoors prevents them from getting too large before they start flowering. The plants can be placed in garden soil where they do very well or they can be grown in containers. Five to 20 gallon containers are suitable. The plants growing in the larger containers will produce more bud.

Marijuana plants can be pruned to keep them a manageable size and help them fit into the garden design. When the main stem is cut, the lower branches enlarge, and the plant grows several strong branches. When these are pruned the plant grows bushier and puts less energy into growing taller. The total yield from a plant with the main stem clipped is greater than its yield when it is unclipped.

Fertilize the plant with a vegetable fertilizer mix or liquid, or use hydroponic vegetative formula to maximize plant growth and yield. Follow directions or use less fertilizer than suggested. Don't use more.

In late summer the lengthening nights trigger the plant to flower. Some varieties cease growing vegetatively almost immediately but others continue growing and quadruple in size. Once the plant starts flowering it usually takes 55-70 days for the buds to mature. When the plant starts flowering, switch the fertilizer to a bloom formula. This will give the plants the nutrients they require to grow big buds, the part of the plant that is harvested and used.

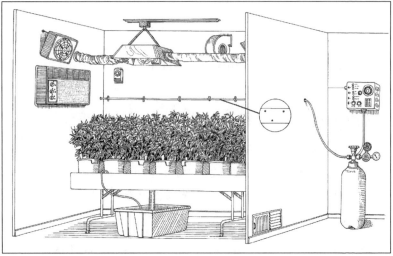

Indoor garden set-up. Courtesy: *Closet Cultivator*

Marijuana plants switch to flowering when the uninterrupted dark period exceeds the critical time period. Critical time varies by variety and is usually between 8 and 11 hours. Plants that respond to a shorter dark period are early season varieties and plants that respond to a longer dark period are late season varieties. If growing outdoors, plants with a short dark period are best suited to higher latitudes.

Marijuana plants must be matched to the latitude because of day length differences between high and low latitude locations. For instance on June 22, the longest day and shortest night of the year, dusk to dawn lasts 8 hours and 44 minutes in San Diego, 8 hours and 3 minutes in St. Louis, and 7 hours and 32 minutes in Boston. Night length is 1 hour and 12 minutes shorter in Boston than in San Diego.

An early season variety growing at low latitudes will be induced to flower early in the season and will remain small even as it matures. The shorter nights during the summer at high latitudes gives the plant a chance to grow before it flowers. A late season variety growing in the north may trigger late in the season and not get a chance to develop mature buds. It will not trigger during the early summer in low latitudes but with the longer nights it flowers earlier in a milder climate.

Marijuana's flowering habits, and the many varieties that have been adapted for specific environmental conditions, have led to many strategies for growing. In northern areas, short season varieties are needed so that plants mature before the weather turns.

In the south, gardeners grow long season varieties during the summer that ripen in the fall. Some short season varieties will start to flower soon, a month after the summer solstice, and will be ready for harvest early in the fall. If not provided with light to extend the day length, many short season varieties will not grow large enough to harvest much of a yield. Long season varieties can be planted in the fall to mature a few months after planting.

In areas that stay warm throughout the year sativas and sativa-indica varieties can be planted in the fall. They will continue to grow in the winter as they flower. They will be ready about 70 to 80 days after placing them in the ground.

No matter what latitude you live in, plants can be triggered to flower at any time during the summer by covering them during a portion of each day so that the night period is lengthened. For instance, if civil dusk is 8:00 p.m., the garden must remain in darkness until 8:00 a.m. By placing an opaque covering over the garden during the dark period and removing it at 8:00 a.m., the plants will receive only 12 hours of light each day and will be triggered into flowering.

Around the sixth week of flowering you will notice that the buds are becoming more odoriferous each day. The unpollinated flowers are beginning to mature. In two or three weeks the flowers will be ripe and ready: the stigma dries, the ovary swells, and

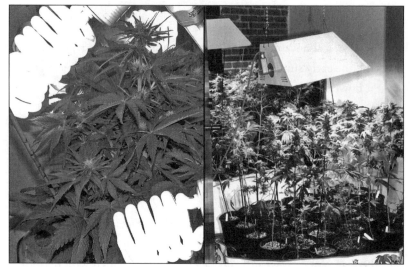

Lighting options: CFLs and HPS. *Photos courtesy of **Marijuana Buds for Less** [left] and **Easy Marijuana Gardening** [right].*

finally the capitate trichomes swell with resin and fluoresce. The bud is ripe. Usually the buds that get the most light ripen first. Remove them but leave the unripe buds to ripen on the plant. They will be ready within 10 days.

Growing Indoors

Indoors, the gardener must supply the plant with all of the things that nature provides outdoors: a planting medium and space large enough for the roots, light, air circulation and satisfactory temperature as well as water and nutrients. Unless your indoor garden space is very bright and gets direct light most of the day, such as from an unobstructed south facing window, the plants will have to be energized using electric lights.

The Size of the Garden

Some gardeners use fluorescent or compact fluorescent lights, but most gardeners use 400, 600 or 1000-watt high pressure so-

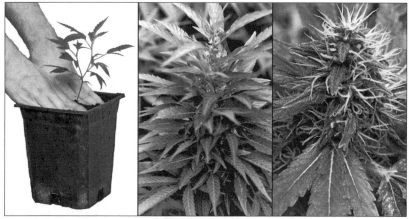

From seedling to bud *Photos: Ed Rosenthal, Seemorebuds (far right)*

dium lamps, which are available on the internet and at indoor garden shops. These lamps require special ballasts, which are included as part of the unit that also includes a reflector.

Plants use light to combine elements in water and carbon dioxide to make sugar and release oxygen. Sugar is the building block for tissue growth- including bud growth, and is used to power metabolism the life process. The more light energy the plant receives and can utilize, the faster and more vigorous the growth. Given the same space, a garden grown under a 400-watt lamp will produce only 40% of the bud than a 1000-watt lamp. Gardens generally yield 3/8-1 gram per watt of lighting. A gardener growing under a single 400-watt lamp can expect to harvest between 6 and 14 ounces every two to four months. Under a 1000-watt lamp the harvest increases to between 13 ounces and 2¼ lbs.

Depending on the variety, plants require between 45 and 60 watts input per square foot of canopy. A 400-watt light illuminates between 6 and 10 square feet; a 1000-watt lamp illuminates between 16 and 20 square feet. Indicas and indica hybrids require less light than sativas and sativa hybrids.

To control temperature in the space, the heat produced by the lights must be removed. Two best ways are to use either an air- or water-cooled reflector. These units enclose the lamp in a cooling system that is separate from the grow space. The air or water is free of odor, because it is inside a tube, so it can be used for heat in another space.

In addition to the heat that the lamp produces, the temperature in the room builds up from the absorption of light, much of which is converted to heat. At the same time the humidity builds up and the CO_2 is quickly mined from the air by the plants. Without more CO_2 the plants cannot produce sugars and growth stops until it is replenished. For all of these reasons the growing space needs to be ventilated with fresh air.

Ventilation can be as easy as opening a curtain or door, or more complex using flexible tubing and an inline fan. Sometimes the ventilation line is controlled by a thermostat/humidistat but some growers keep the ventilation going whenever the lights are on.

Indoor gardeners have a choice of whether to grow in planting containers with planting mix or to use hydroponics. Hydroponic systems use a non-nutritive rooting medium and provide nutrients by adding fertilizer to the water. Hydroponics requires a bit more skill and a higher degree of accuracy because there are no natural buffers in the medium. It will not be covered in this section, but there are many books on the subject.

Whether you are starting with sexed seedlings or clones, the plants should be grown in containers filled with a high quality, enriched indoor planting mix. Three-gallon containers are a convenient size to use. They aren't too heavy, they give the roots room to grow and they will support a plant with a diameter of about two square feet.

Clip the top bit of growth of the center stem when you transplant the young plants. Keep the lights on 18-24 hours a day.

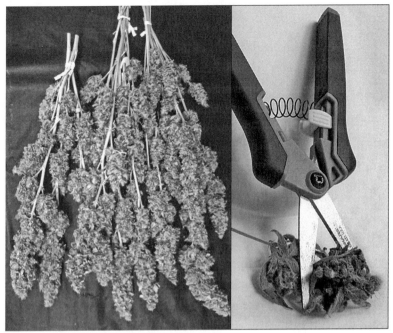

Harvest and manicuring, *Photos: Ed Rosenthal*

The longer the light is on each day the faster the plants will grow to flowering size.

After three weeks the plants should be 1-1½ feet (30 to 45 cm) tall and ready to flower. Change the light cycle to 12 hours dark and 12 hours light. Use a timer so the light goes on and off at the same time each day. Don't interrupt the dark period even momentarily with light. The only kind of light that is safe to use in the dark garden is a green light, which doesn't affect the plant. Change the fertilizer to a flowering formula. In 7-10 weeks depending on the variety the top buds will be ripe. Buds underneath the top canopy should be left on the plant. They will ripen in 7-10 days.

Manicuring

Once the buds are cut they should be manicured. All the large leaves and the smaller leaves are trimmed off. Only the tiny leaves and the flowers are left. Then the buds are placed on a tray or hung to dry in a cool area with good ventilation and air circulation. A closet, spare room or basement area might be suitable. Depending on the humidity, the buds will dry in 5 to 10 days. The buds are considered dry when the small stems holding them together snaps firmly when it is bent.

The leaf that was trimmed away should be dried so it can be used for cooking or to make kief, which is the screened glands, separated from the leaf tissue.

Once they have dried to stem crack, it is time to trim the buds from the stem. Place them in a glass jar and close it. If the buds begin to "sweat," that is, if there are any signs of moisture, open the lid and let it evaporate. This may occur a few times over the first few days. When the buds stop sweating they are ready to use.

Chapter 6
Preparation and Dosage Methods

Potency of Plants and Plant Parts

Earlier, we mentioned briefly that different varieties and even different plants of the same variety vary in potency. Usually, domestic marijuana contains a higher proportion of THC than Mexican varieties, which are mostly grown outdoors and not cultivated as sinsemilla. However, since the early 1990s, higher-quality Canadian "BC Bud," consisting of indoor-grown sinsemilla, has been imported in large quantities.

Environmental factors play a part in the potency of the bud. Growing conditions, weather, and care affect the quality of marijuana, just as with flowers and vegetables.

Different parts of the marijuana plant have different potencies. THC is found in glands that grow on the surface of the plant's stem and leaves. These resin-exuding glands, known as trichomes, resemble miniature mushrooms under the microscope. The Trichomes are most concentrated on the tiny leaves and stems surrounding and inside the clusters of female flowers. Larger leaves from this area are usually picked off (manicured) once the buds have been harvested. These leaves are called trim. They contain less THC than the smaller leaves and organs surrounding the flower. The large fan or sun leaves contain even fewer glands and are considerably less potent than the flowers or the trim.

Drug warriors have tried to scare the public about the supposed hazards of more potent marijuana. They ignore the advantages of higher-potency marijuana for reducing smoke inhalation. Federal officials have claimed that the potency of marijuana has increased so drastically that it is effectively a whole new drug. In fact, however, the range of potencies available has not changed over the years. High-potency preparations, including hashish, hash oil, special strains, and extracts have been widely available since the nineteenth century. However, it is true that the average potency of marijuana has increased somewhat due to increasing use of higher-quality indoor sinsemilla.

High-potency formulations have a long tradition of medical use. Up through the 1930s, when cannabis was available over the counter in pharmacies throughout the U.S., it was sold in alcohol-based tinctures of 25% potency. Recommended doses were measured in drops.

On balance, high-potency sinsemilla and concentrated preparations are preferable for most medical users to protect them from harmful smoke. When inhalation is not necessary, oral ingestion is better.

Concentrating Grass

Sinsemilla [from the Spanish *sin*, "without" and *semilla*, "seeds"] marijuana buds retail for hundreds of dollars per ounce—up to several thousand dollars per pound—and usually contain between 4% and 20% THC. The large fan leaves contain between 2% and 3% THC; they retail for only $100 to $300 per pound. The trim leaves contain 2% to 3% THC and retail for $200 to $500 per pound. You can see that the leaves and trim are much more economical than the buds and are truly the best buy. The only problem is that they are harsh on the throat and not pleasant to smoke.

The solution to this dilemma is to concentrate the THC so that only the potent part—the glands—is used. There are several ways to do this.

Screening

The easiest screen to use is a silkscreen or, even better, a steel or plastic mesh screen with 100 or 125 lines to the inch. The spaces in the screen are large enough to allow the glands to drop through. Suitable framed screens are available at marijuana dispensaries or through the Internet. The vegetable material stays on the top. The yield depends on the quality of the material you started with.

To use a screen, first dry the marijuana by placing it in a microwave oven. The marijuana is dry enough to screen when it crumbles or snaps in the hand. It need not be broken up. Placed the dried marijuana in a freezer until it is thoroughly chilled. This will make it easier to remove the glands.

If you're using a screen made of silk or other fine cloth, stretch it tight over a collection vessel (such as a bowl). Framed screens may simply be placed over a table or tray. Rub the dried, chilled plant material over the screen. The longer the material is rubbed, the more glands will fall through. Note, however, that longer rubbings also increase the amount of plant debris that comes through the screen. The process is analogous to olive pressing, in which the longer the press, the lower the quality of the oil, because more impurities are pressed out.

Concentrating cannabis by screening requires a little finesse and practice. The end use that you have in mind can help you decide when to stop screening. The very first screening produces the best 'kief'–unpressed hashish. Glands that fall through the screen can be smoked in a pipe, added to a joint, or ingested. They are extremely potent, so only a little bit is needed. Excess plant debris makes the screened cannabis less desirable for smoking, but the additional vegetative matter is not as significant when the pot is eaten. So for smoking, aim for the purest resin you can get. For eating, a larger yield, even if in a less concentrated form, is the goal.

Water Screening

THC glands are heavier than water and sink, whereas most vegetative material is lighter and floats. This makes it easy to concentrate the glands as long as they can be detached from the vegetative material. The resulting "kief" is very clean and concentrated. Before water screening, the grass can be screened mechanically, but it doesn't have to be. Since the glands are literally washed, pollutants, molds, and fungi are rinsed away.

Whole marijuana is put in a jar. Cold water and a few ice cubes are added. Then the mix is shaken for a few minute or so. The vegetative material stays on top and is removed. The THC-containing glands fall to the bottom. They are rinsed out of the jar and dried.

Don't use warm or even tepid water. With ice-cold water, the glands remain rigid and brittle. When warm water is used, they become soft and sticky; this makes them much harder to work with.

The glands are very powerful. Only a pinch is needed in a pipe bowl to provide relief. They can also be swallowed in capsules or eaten in food.

One medical user uses the THC-bearing glands in cooking. She has a small container of the substance and uses a tiny spoon to add it to her food.

Methods of Taking the Dose

Cannabis can be smoked or vaporized, used as a tincture, ingested, or used topically. Each method of use has its advantages and disadvantages. The different methods can be used separately or together.

Inhaled THC: Smoking and vaporization

Smoking is the most common way people use marijuana. It takes little equipment and is very fast-acting. THC in inhaled smoke takes only a few seconds to reach the user's bloodstream. Its effects can be felt as soon as it reaches the receptors in the brain and organs, usually in less than a minute. The main drawback to smoking is, of course, the smoke. Cannabis smoke has some (though not all) of the same toxins as cigarette smoke. Some users find smoke of any kind difficult to tolerate.

Vaporization is a healthier alternative to smoking. It allows users to inhale the THC and cannabinoids without the toxic tars and gases in the smoke, while offering the same benefits of rapid delivery as smoking. However vaporization takes a bit more in the way of hardware than smoking. There are many commercial vaporizers available, and users can find instructions for building their own online. Also, users who are accustomed to smoking cannabis may need to get used to the different feel of the vaporizer, which is much subtler and lighter than the smoke from a joint or pipe.

Whether smoked or vaporized, inhaled THC gives a very characteristic user experience. Once it takes effect, the high grows quickly for about 15 minutes then deepens a little for another 10 to 20 minutes. After this peak, the high begins to fade and is gone within one to three hours. This helps relieve symptoms quickly. The rapid effect also makes it easier to determine how much to use. Patients suffering from nausea or loss of appetite find that inhalation offers special advantages for them, as they don't have to eat it.

Both the individual's susceptibility to marijuana and the marijuana quality affect the high. Lower-quality marijuana is felt as quickly as high-quality, but it reaches its peak more quickly and lasts a shorter time.

Tinctures: an alternative to smoking

A tincture is a concentrated extract of marijuana, usually prepared in a base of alcohol, oil, or glycerol. This method offers a middle ground between inhalation and ingestion. Tinctures are used under the tongue, or sublingually. They are quickly absorbed through the mucus membranes in the patient's mouth. Then they migrate directly to the bloodstream–bypassing the liver, which becomes involved in oral ingestion. The effects are felt in five minutes or less, and the high then develops very much like that from inhaled THC.

Taking THC in a tincture is a good substitute method for patients who are uncomfortable with smoking. It is almost as fast-acting as inhalation, requires only a bottle and an eyedropper, and can be less conspicuous than smoking as there is no smoke or smell. Tinctures may be purchased directly from a dispensary or prepared at home. [*See Chapter 7, Cooking with Marijuana.*]

Ingestion: Marijuana as food

Ingestion produces somewhat different effects from inhalation because anything absorbed through the stomach is processed by the liver before it reaches the brain. In the liver, THC is converted to 11-hydroxy-THC, a metabolite that is if anything more psychoactive than ordinary THC. Because 11-hydroxy-THC is not produced when marijuana is smoked, eating and smoking produce different pharmacological effects.

Ingested marijuana takes longer to be felt and its effects last longer. The long-lasting nature of ingested marijuana can be very helpful for some patients. Some people regulate their conditions by eating small amounts of marijuana on a regular basis, sometimes just once or twice a day. They barely feel any effect from the drug except for the relief of their symptoms. Of course the slow onset is a drawback when a patient needs immediate relief for acute symptoms.

One of the advantages of ingestion is that it works well with relatively low-grade marijuana, such as leaf. Because leaf is considered a by-product of bud production it tends to be inexpensive and readily available. This material can be dried and ground as "leaf flour" and used in a variety of recipes (including marijuana butter or oil used in cooking).

The major drawback of ingesting marijuana is that the effective dose can be difficult to predict. Depending on the state of your digestive system, the contents of your stomach, and other hard to measure factors, a given oral dose may be absorbed more or less easily. It also may take several hours to take full effect. This makes it difficult to know beforehand how much to eat.

Topical Use

Some patients apply marijuana externally, or topically, to the skin in the form of ointments, lotions, or poultices, for treatment of swollen joints and skin inflammation. Laboratory studies by a team at the University of Bonn, Germany, found that topical applications of THC helped mice heal faster from skin allergies [Karsak[1]].

It's not clear how topical treatment works. Indeed, many researchers believe there is no effective method for transporting THC or other cannabinoids through the skin. Dr. Mahmoud ElSohly, who directs NIDA's marijuana research garden, has proposed using rectal suppositories, which he claims are a better way of delivering cannabinoids to the system. Other investigators claim to have developed topical cannabinoids that penetrate the skin, but their products haven't been independently tested and aren't commercially available.

Still, many patients claim they find benefits in direct application. Tom claimed that his rheumatoid arthritis was relieved by rubbing his joints with an ointment made from 4 ounces of marijuana leaf soaked in 16 ounces of oil. He applied the ointment with alcohol. Marijuana-based salves have traditionally been used in Mexico for muscle and joint pains.

It is possible that topical preparations don't deliver cannabinoids but other, more soluble, medically active ingredients, such as terpenoids or flavonoids, through the skin. Topical cannabis extracts were shown to have anti-inflammatory properties in laboratory animal experiments by E.A. Formukong at the University of London School of Pharmacy. [Formukong[2]]

---

1 Karsak M, et al, "Attenuation of Allergic Contact Dermatitis Through the Endocannabinoid System," Science 316:1494-97 (2007).
2 Formukong EA, Evans AT, and Evans FJ, "Analgesic and antiinflammatory activity of constitutents of Cannabis sativa L," Inflammation 12(4):361 (1988).

At the turn of the century, cannabis was used as a topical ingredient in remedies for corns (either as an anesthetic or as a coloring agent). Topical cannabis applications are also used in folk medicine in India and Latin America. One popular treatment for arthritis in the Mexican-American community is to wrap the joints in a poultice, or bandage, of cannabis leaves. In order to promote extraction of the cannabinoids, the leaves are soaked in alcohol.

Killing Pathogens in Marijuana

Many doctors recommend that patients with impaired immune systems sterilize all marijuana that they use, whether it's smoked or eaten. They may be saying this as a matter of course rather than because there is a real danger of infection. However, a few people have become sick from infected marijuana. In particular, there have been reports of aspergillosis, a lung infection caused by inhalation of spores from the aspergillus fungus, which is particularly dangerous to HIV patients.[3]

Aspergillus and other pathogens require moisture to grow. Controlling dampness is therefore key to preventing contamination. Marijuana should be dried to around 10%–15% water content in order to prevent fungal growth (below 10% it becomes too brittle). A stale or moldy smell is a sign of likely contamination.

In practice, it's difficult to know whether marijuana has become contaminated, especially if one hasn't overseen every step in its preparation. Sterilization is therefore advisable to kill any pathogens. One might expect any pathogens to die in the burn when marijuana is smoked. However, the smoke does pass through cooler, unburned material, so pathogens can enter the smoke stream.

---

3 Hamadeh, R et al, "Fatal aspergillosis associated with smoking contaminated marijuana, in a marrow transplant recipient," Chest 94:432-33 (1988); Llamas, R, et al, "Allergenic bronchopulmonary aspergillosis associated with moldy marijuana." Chest 73:871-872 (1978).

Though the chance of infection is low, it's best for people with injured immune systems to make sure that pathogens are killed before they use marijuana. The most practical method for doing this is to heat the marijuana. Baking in a home oven at a temperature of 300° F (150° C) for five minutes is sufficient to destroy aspergillus. Be careful not to overheat the marijuana, since THC will vaporize at higher temperatures. A more high-tech method is gamma irradiation, which is used to sterilize the medical marijuana produced by the Netherlands.

Marijuana will occasionally become visibly moldy. Mold can grow while the marijuana is in the field, if it is packed without proper drying, or if it stored in damp conditions. Such mold will be readily visible when the marijuana is unpacked. The marijuana is unusable at that point even if the mold is killed, because fungal toxins will remain and cannot be removed.

Preparing Marijuana for Smoking

The "ripe" marijuana bud is the part of the plant that is used for smoking. To burn evenly and smoke well, properly prepared bud should be free of sticks and seeds because these produce a harsh, unpleasant smoke. Marijuana leaf is seldom smoked because of its low potency and its harsh "dry" smoke. Instead, leaf is used mainly in processed products.

Most domestically grown marijuana is sinsemilla, that is, seedless. Most imported marijuana, such as Mexican, contains a considerable number of seeds. These must be removed before the marijuana is smoked, or they will pop when they get hot. This can send a hard-burning particle, or at least a very hot one, in any direction, but usually toward the most recent clothing purchase that is in the immediate area. Burning seed also releases an acrid smoke that most people find foul. Some even find that burning seed gives them a mild headache.

The best way to remove seeds from marijuana is to break several marijuana buds up by cutting them with a pair of scissors, so that all the seeds are released from the vegetation. Remove any small twigs at this stage. Don't try to remove the seeds at this point, though; it will be too tedious.

Most people use their fingers to remove the seeds from their bud, but when they do this many of the resin glands are broken off and stick to the skin, removing some of the active ingredient. After the first layer of glands has stuck to the skin, glands that they come in contact with also stick. This is all right if you're manicuring large amounts. After a while, a layer builds up that is thick enough to be rubbed off the fingers. This mixture of glands and human oils is a form of hashish and can be smoked. Since it is a concentration of the glands, it is much more potent than the buds.

If you're cleaning only enough for a few joints, however, only a thin layer of glands builds up. It does not easily peel or rub off the skin, although it's easily removed using a tissue or soap and water. Either way, it's lost.

There is a partial solution. Use scissors to cut the buds up. Not as many glands will stick to the scissors as to your fingers. The glands accumulate on the scissors and can eventually be scraped off. Still, many of the glands never make it to the joint.

Removing the seeds from marijuana is best done using a "rolling tray," which can be as simple as a shoe-box top, a plate, or a screen device. You place the grass at one end of the tray. The tray is held at a slight angle, with the grass at the lower end, and using a business card, a playing card (not the Queen of Spades), or a canceled credit card, you push the vegetation and seeds toward the top, up the slope. The heavy, slightly oval seeds will roll down while the vegetation stays in place. Continue doing this until the seeds stop rolling out. Then look for any seeds that may be hidden and gently nudge them to start them rolling. When all the seeds have been removed, the marijuana is ready to use.

Sinsemilla is handled differently. Since there are no seeds, the buds don't need to be broken up for cleaning. They need only be cut or ground finely enough to roll into a joint or place in the bowl of a pipe. If you use a photographer's loupe, you can see the glands on the surfaces of the buds and leaves. The heads of these glands contain the THC. Be aware that these glands break away from the leaf at the slightest provocation, such as a touch or even a strong wind. This lowers the amount left to use.

METHODS OF SMOKING
Joints

Joints (marijuana cigarettes) are probably the most common way people smoke marijuana. They are convenient to use, are easy to carry and dispose of, leave no paraphernalia trail, and are easily shared. Many people get oral satisfaction from toking on a joint in the same way as they might if smoking a cigarette.

Before marijuana can be rolled into a joint, it must be broken into small pieces so that it will be evenly distributed. This is easily done using scissors. Economical, hand-held herb grinders are also available for processing sinsemilla.

Joints can be rolled using a hand rolling machine or completely by hand. They're rolled different ways. The two that are most familiar to us are the American joint and the Dutch spliff. People who have difficulty hand-rolling joints can use one of the ma-

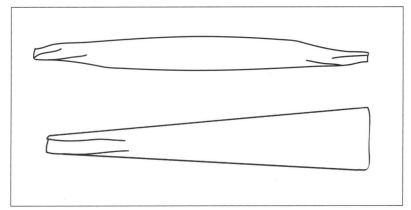

Regular (top) and European (bottom) joint

chine rollers available in some smoke shops. Joints come in many sizes. A joint is smoked much like a cigarette. The smoker draws air through the joint so that the airstream picks up the smoke.

Pipes

Pipes have grown in popularity and many people prefer them to joints. There are several reasons. Unlike joints, they use no paper or glue, so the smoke contains no impurities. They usually have small bowls that allow the user to use just enough bud for a single toke. This prevents waste from sidestream smoke (the smoke that rises constantly from the end of a burning joint). Pipes also avoid the waste of bud when a joint becomes too short to hold or smoke.

There are innumerable pipe designs, ranging from the most basic implements to true works of art. No matter how stylish the pipe is, it should have an easy draw, be comfortable to use, and be easy to clean.

Pipes have been made from every conceivable material and innumerable designs. In a pipe shop, you're likely to see glass, wood, metal, and plastic pipes, ranging from purely functional implements to true works of art. But no matter the variations, any good pipe should be comfortable to use, easy to clean, and have a smooth, easy draw.

Materials are mostly a matter of personal preference. There have been no studies specifically checking residues from heated pipes, but it is generally agreed that glass, ceramic, stainless steel, and brass are inert. Burning wood may produce some fumes, but hardwoods require a greater heat than that in the bowl to start smoldering. Avoid plastic pipes. No matter the maker's claims, plastic is better suited for blowing bubbles than holding hot coals.

Some pipes feature a "carburetor," which is a small hole in the air chamber located past the bowl. The carburetor is held shut while the bowl is being lit and the smoke drawn. Then, when the carburetor is released, the smoke is drawn into the lungs more quickly.

Waterpipes and Bongs

As the name suggests, waterpipes work by drawing the smoke through a reservoir of water. This both cools the smoke and removes particles from it, making the draw smoother. Just as with conventional pipes, people have applied tremendous ingenuity to the design of waterpipes. There are an incredible number of styles and designs.

Most pipes have a bowl on top of a stem that ends below the waterline. The air tube is above the water. When you draw on the tube, air is pulled through the bowl, the stem, and the water, so the water filters the smoke. The smaller the size of the bubbles and the greater the length of the tube of water through which they pass, the more filtering the water does.

A bong is a specialized type of waterpipe; it has a large chamber in which the smoke is held before it is inhaled, and a carburetor hole similar to those on some regular pipes. When the carburetor is released, a large amount of smoke can be inhaled quickly.

Although many folks prefer to use waterpipes because of the cooler, smoother smoke they produce, there's no evidence that waterpipes are actually healthier for the lungs. One problem is that waterpipes tend to absorb even more THC than they do other, carcinogenic compounds. As a result, users may end up consuming more harmful smoke toxins in order to absorb the same dose of THC.

A smoking device study, sponsored by California NORML and MAPS (the Multidisciplinary Association for Psychedelic Studies), found that waterpipes absorb more cannabinoids than carcinogenic tars [Gieringer[4]]. Therefore, in order to obtain the same effective dose of THC, a smoker would end up taking in at least 30% more tars from a waterpipe than from an unfiltered joint. The more thorough the water filtration, the lower the proportion of THC to total tars, and the greater the amount of THC wasted by absorption in the pipe water.

Nonetheless, the study did not examine the vapor phase of the smoke, which contains numerous toxic gases, such as carbon monoxide, aldehydes, phenols, and hydrogen cyanide. Some of these are quite water soluble, and therefore likely to be screened out by waterpipes. If so, waterpipes could have significant health benefits. Further research is needed to determine whether waterpipes are on balance counterproductive or helpful.

A more dubious smoke filtration strategy is to inhale the smoke through a cigarette filter. Though there are a number of ingenious devices to accomplish this, they offer no advantages. The NORML-MAPS study found that cigarette filters had the same

---

4 Gieringer D, "The California/MAPS Smoking Device Study," MAPS Newsletter 1996; http://www.canorml.org/healthfacts/smokestudy.html.

drawbacks as waterpipes, increasing the ratio of tars to THC by some 30%. Unlike waterpipes, there is no reason to expect that cigarette filters would reduce toxic gases. Worst of all, though, the study found that they eliminated fully 60% of the THC from the smoke stream. This means you would have to smoke 2.5 times as much marijuana through a cigarette filter to get the same dose of THC as with an unfiltered joint!

Vaporizers

By far the best method for avoiding toxic smoke is to use a vaporizer. Vaporizers heat marijuana to a temperature below the point of combustion–around 356°–392° F (180° – 200° C), where the medically active components of the resin evaporate without any toxic smoke or burning. The vapor is then inhaled, delivering a smooth, clean, effective dosage of cannabinoids without any smoke or combustion byproducts. Vaporization works because the medically active cannabinoids and terpenes reside in resin on the external surface of the leaf trichomes, and these components vaporize below the ignition point of the plant matter. Following vaporization, the leftover marijuana is dried and crisp, but

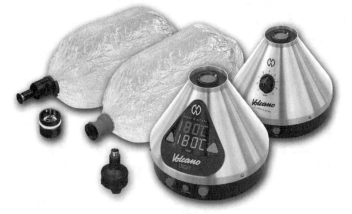

Volcano vaporizer

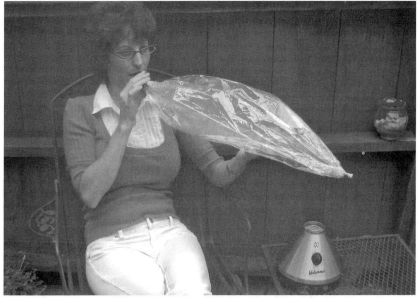

Angel Raich using a Volcano vaporizer. Raich's lawsuit to let her use marijuana for an inoperable brain tumor and other life-threatening conditions was rejected by the U.S. Supreme Court.

retains its shape and has a greenish-brown hue. In contrast, combusted marijuana disintegrates into black and gray ashes.

The technology of vaporization has progressed rapidly since the first edition of this book was published ten years ago. At that time, the technology was still unproven, and commercial models weren't readily available. Since then, new research has confirmed the effectiveness of vaporizers, and numerous models have reached the market.

In a study sponsored by California NORML and MAPS [Gieringer[5]], a vaporizer known as the M-1 Volatizer® was found to effectively deliver THC while completely eliminating three known toxic hydrocarbons – benzene, toluene, and naphthalene – from the vapor. The study also found substantially reduced carbon monoxide emissions, but did not test for other chemicals. The M-1 (see photo) consisted of an electric heater designed to

5 Gieringer D, "Cannabis Vaporization: A Promising Strategy for Smoke Harm Reduction," Journal of Cannabis Therapeutics, 1(3/4):153-70 (2001).

fit over a pipe bowl and radiate heat downwards into the sample. This is not necessarily the best design, since it tends to overheat the surface nearest the heat and underheat the lower layers.

A more exhaustive follow-up study was conducted using a more advanced vaporization device: the Volcano®, manufactured by Storz & Bickel of Tuttlingen, Germany [Gieringer[6]]. The Volcano® includes an automatic temperature control, an air blower to facilitate even heating of the sample, and a vapor collection balloon. The study found that the Volcano emitted vapors consisting overwhelmingly of THC, whereas the smoke from combusted marijuana consisted of 100 other chemicals, including carcinogenic polycyclic aromatic hydrocarbons.

Dr. Donald Abrams at the University of California at San Francisco subsequently tested the Volcano in human subjects [Abrams et al.[7]]. The study examined the amount of THC delivered to the bloodstream via vaporization and smoking. The Volcano® was shown to deliver a consistent dosage of THC to the subjects, with an efficiency somewhat greater than smoked marijuana. The increased efficiency may be explained by the fact that some THC is destroyed in combustion. Abrams' study also found lower levels of carbon monoxide gas in subjects who used the vaporizer. Abrams' study effectively validated the use of vaporizers in medical research. Given the strong medical opposition to the use of smoked medications, vaporization is apt to be the way of the future for cannabis medicine.

Many kinds of vaporizers are presently available on the market. Because paraphernalia laws still prohibit devices for administering marijuana, they are legally sold for use as "herbal vaporizers"

---

6 Gieringer D and St. Laurent J, "Cannabis Vaporizer Combines Efficient Delivery of THC With Effective Suppression Of Pyrolytic Compounds" Journal of Cannabis Therapeutics Vol. 4 #1 (2004).

7 Abrams D, et al, "Vaporization as a Smokeless Cannabis Delivery System: A Pilot Study", Clinical Pharmacology and Therapeutics 82(5) 2007; pp 572-78.

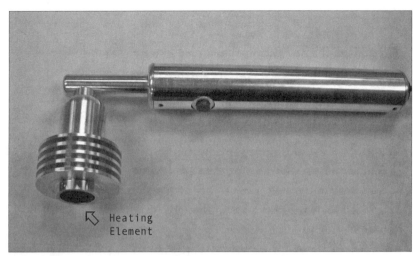

M-1 Volatizer: Heating element is placed over pipe bowl.

(vaporization works on many other medicinal herbs, as well as tobacco). A web search for vaporizers will turn up scores of devices, selling for prices ranging from $20 to $500. At the high end is the Volcano, which currently ranks as the Rolls Royce of vaporizers, as well as the only one tested in medical studies. At the other end of the spectrum, one can buy inexpensive, portable, hand-held glass vaporization tubes, which are supposed to be stuffed with marijuana and heated externally to the proper temperature by a hand-held cigarette lighter. The problem with such designs is that it is difficult to maintain the proper level of heat consistently with a hand-held flame. All too frequently, either the sample is overheated and scorched, or else it is underheated and a significant amount of medicine is left unvaporized.

Even, controllable heat is one of the most important considerations when shopping for a vaporizer. Avoid models that use direct contact to heat the sample. This tends to overheat the marijuana nearest the heating element while leaving the more distant material underheated. This was a common design problem in the earliest vaporizers and many homemade models, which heated the marijuana on a hot plate or through the walls of a heating chamber. The best way to obtain even heating is to force heated air through the sample using a blower.

Another important vaporizer feature is a reliable, automatic temperature control. It's hard to maintain good results if you must constantly adjust the heat by hand using eyeball judgments.

A final consideration is convenience and portability. A major disadvantage of the Volcano – as well as most other vaporizers–is its need for an electric outlet. The race is on to develop good, portable, rechargeable devices.

Use High-Potency Marijuana

In the absence of high-tech smoking devices, the easiest way to reduce noxious smoke toxins is simply to use stronger pot. More potent material reduces your exposure to harmful tars simply by requiring less smoke to get the same dose of THC. Theoretically, high-grade sinsemilla with a potency of 12% should deliver six times as much THC per puff as low-grade "ditchweed" with a potency of 2%. In practice, this may not be entirely accurate. Researchers have found that high-potency grades do not necessarily deliver THC as effectively as low-grade leaf, perhaps because of inefficient burning [Gowing et al.[8]]. On the other hand, there are some hash oil extracts that are so potent that a single toke can be more than enough. It's therefore important to be careful in experimenting with extremely high-potency varieties.

---

8 Gowing L, et al, "Respiratory Harms of Smoked Cannabis," Drug and Alcohol Services Council of South Australia, DASC Monograph 8, July 2000.

Chapter 7
Cooking with Marijuana

Cooking with Bud, Hash, or Kief

Most of the recipes in this section assume that you'll be using cannabis leaf. Leaf is the best value for cooking with pot, because it gives you the most bang for the buck. However sometimes you'll have something more potent on hand such as bud, hashish, or kief. Hash especially is very traditional in many pot recipes (possibly because it has less of the "weedy" taste found in some leaf). If you want to use the more potent pot preparations in your recipes then use these conversion factors to control your dose:

For 1 ounce of regular domestic leaf called for in the recipe, use:

+ 0.25-0.5 ounce (6-15 grams) of medium-grade sinsemilla buds

+ 0.125-0.25 ounce (3-7 grams) of high-grade sinsemilla buds

+ 3-4 grams of hash or best-quality sinsemilla buds

Ingestion

Eating marijuana is a very pleasant way to take it as medicine. Unlike the immediate sensation you feel when you smoke it, the effect comes on more gradually, beginning about 20 to 30 minutes on an empty stomach, to an hour or longer after heavy eating.

The problem with eating marijuana is that its effects tend to be unpredictable. Depending on the state of your digestive system, the THC may or may not be well absorbed, so the same dose may be too much or too little. In addition, the potency of edibles is hard to gauge beforehand. Different recipes, batches, and ingredients can yield wildly different results, and DEA regulations forbid commercial potency testing of cannabis edibles.

Once the effects begin, they usually peak within an hour, remain at that level for one and one-half to two hours, and then diminish over the next hour or two. To avoid a sharp peak in effects, some people nibble on the medicine rather than eat it all at once. They might eat as little as 10% of their highest dose, then take a bite every 15 or 20 minutes, finishing the portion over the course of several hours.

The amount of time that effects are felt is variable, and depends on whether you have food in your stomach, etc. If you eat marijuana brownies for dessert after a big meal, you may not begin to feel high for 2-3 hours. If you eat the brownie on an empty stomach, the effects will be much quicker.

Since there's a long wait before you feel marijuana's effects after you eat it, trying to find the right amount to use can be frustrating. Probably the simplest way to do this is to eat half the recommended dose. If that doesn't give you relief, wait until the effects have subsided, then try again, increasing the amount by another 10% of the recommended dose. Do this until you find a comfortable level.

Nibbling also reduces the risk of a heavy overdose. When you nibble, you're using only a portion of a large dose at any one time, so the effects never reach the intensity of the full dose at its peak.

THC is oil- and fat-soluble, but does not dissolve well in water. In order to efficiently dissolve the THC, marijuana is best prepared in butter, oil, milk or alcohol.

Lecithin is an ingredient in many marijuana recipes. It is an emulsifier, which means it helps water and oil to mix. It is found in milk, keeping the mixture of oils and water together, as well as in soybeans. It's used commercially in many foods, such as salad dressings. Commercial dressings don't separate right away because the emulsifier causes their component liquids to break up into small bubbles when you shake them. The small bubbles take a longer time to float or sink into position. Lecithin is available in both liquid and dry forms at health food stores. Glycerin is another option for dissolving cannabinoids.

Marijuana Makes Weak Tea

Although some patients like to make tea by steeping marijuana in hot water, this is a notably inefficient use of the plant. Because THC is not water soluble, very little gets mixed into the tea. If marijuana is boiled in hot water for 15 – 30 minutes (the longer the better), a small amount of THC will be left in an oily film floating on top of the water when it cools. Although you can use it without mixing it with oil or alcohol, not as much will pass through the intestines to the bloodstream that way, so its effect won't be as strong.

Furthermore, boiling water is not hot enough to efficiently convert the THC acid (THCA) in the plant into active THC. As we have seen, THCA has little apparent activity, though it might conceivably benefit some patients. A study of cannabis tea from the Netherlands Office of Medicinal Cannabis found that marijuana steeped in boiling water for 15 minutes yielded four times as much THCA as THC. In all, only 5% of the THC was delivered to the water [Hazekamp[1]]. You can strengthen marijuana tea by (1) adding milk or butter to help extract the THC and (2) heating the marijuana beforehand to convert the THCA into active THC.

Preparing Marijuana for Ingestion

In order to make efficient use of marijuana, the THCA in the plant must be converted to its active form via a process known as decarboxylation. The THCA is normally decarboxlyated by heating and drying the plant. This occurs automatically in smoking or at normal stove or oven temperatures in cooking. However, if marijuana is not heated, most of the cannabinoids will remain in their less active acid form. This is especially true for newly harvested, fresh marijuana. Over a period of months, marijuana will gradually decarboxylate when kept dry at room temperature.

If you plan to prepare marijuana without cooking it in the stove or oven, you may want to preheat it beforehand so as to activate the THC. Lab tests have found that THCA can be 100% decarboxylated by heating it to 390° F (200° C) for five minutes. However, since this is above the vaporization temperature of THC (350° F or 180° C), the sample should be protected from evaporation. This can be done by absorbing it in oil or sealing it in foil or an airtight container. In practice, lower temperatures are preferable, both to avoid vaporization and to preserve the flavor of the marijuana, which tends to turn burnt and unsavory when overheated. One effective method is to heat the sample to 212° F (100° C) for ninety minutes. That can be done in a dry oven, or by sealing the

---

1 Hazekamp A, et al, "Cannabis tea revisited: A systematic evaluation of the cannabinoid composition of cannabis tea," Journal of Ethnopharmacology, : 85-90 (2007).

TEMPERATURE EFFECTS ON MARIJUANA

Temperature		Where	Effects on
°F	°C	Found	Marijuana
68-75	20-24	Normal Room Temperature	The most volatile terpenes gradually vaporize, producing characteristic odor.
96-100	35-38	Human Body Temperature	Increased vaporization makes odor stronger and richer.
212	100	Boiling Water	THC-acid is completely decarboxylated after 90 minutes at 100° C dry heat
265-300	130-150	Cool Vaporizer	The most volatile terpenes vaporize completely. THC-acid decarboxylates gradually, but little THC vaporizes.
300	150	Oven	Five minutes at this temperature kills spores of aspergillus fungus. Most terpenes vaporize.
355-400	180-200	Ideal Vaporizer Temperature	Terpenes completely vaporized. About 5%-10% of THC vaporizes in 90 seconds.
445	230	Hot Vaporizer / Oven	THC completely decarboxylates in 5 minutes. About 30% of THC vaporizes in 90 seconds. Marijuana is left dry and crisp.
455+	235+	Flame	Combustion point: marijuana ignites. Terpenes and THC come off in the smoke.

sample in an airtight container and placing it in boiling water or a hot pot. A decarboxylation device known as the Maximizer® used to be commercially available, but was forced off the market by anti-paraphernalia laws in the early 1980s.

Reducing the "Weedy" Flavor of Marijuana

There are some recipes that just don't go well with the strong flavor of marijuana, which comes from its water-soluble compounds. However, these can be extracted, leaving the leaf with a much less intense flavor.

Use the whole leaf. Place the marijuana in a bowl, being sure not to pack it too tightly. Add tepid water and let the marijuana soak for about half an hour. The water changes color as much of the chlorophyll and other pigments are dissolved. Pour off the water. The marijuana is now ready to be used as is, or it can be dried and powdered.

After pouring off the water and removing the marijuana, you'll probably see a tan-colored residue at the bottom of the bowl. This substance consists of glands that have fallen off the leaf. It can be dried and is very potent. This process is similar to the "water screening" process we described earlier.

Dry Preparation (Leaf or Bud Flour)

This is the main preparation method for most of the recipes in this chapter. Unless a recipe states otherwise, it uses marijuana "flour" that has been dried and ground as follows. This process can be used with any form of marijuana–buds, trim, or leaf. The marijuana may have gone through the water process described above or not, but it must be very dry.

Marijuana is ground using a blender. First the marijuana is dried until it is crisp and breaks easily in your fingers. This can be done in a microwave oven or a food dehydrator. Sensitive ovens with a setting of 100 degrees Fahrenheit (38 degrees Centigrade) also work well. Once the marijuana is dry, place it in a blender on high speed. If only a small amount is being processed, a coffee grinder may be more convenient. Grind the marijuana until it is powdery. Don't open the top right away, because the dust, which contains the THC-bearing glands, has to settle first. This takes about five minutes.

Once it has been ground, the marijuana is sifted through a strainer. This is done to remove unchopped leaf veins. It should be done in a room with little air circulation, using a high-walled bowl, not a plate, so that the ultra-light THC glands don't drift into the atmosphere. Once the marijuana is ground and sifted, it is ready to use in cooking.

Alcohol, Glycerin, or Oil Extract Preparation

The most popular way of cooking with grass is to dissolve the THC in drinkable alcohol, butter, or oil. This can be done after soaking the marijuana in water. The color of the alcohol, butter, or oil doesn't become as deep and the flavor doesn't get as intense.

Making an alcohol mix is very easy. Just add the grass to any 80-proof or stronger beverage alcohol. The theory is that the stronger the alcohol, the more THC will be dissolved in it. Though this theory has not been tested, we suspect that 80-proof (40%) alcohol is strong enough to dissolve all the THC. Most of the THC dissolves within a few hours. Within two days, the process is complete. Mixing or shaking the alcohol helps this process along.

DO NOT use rubbing alcohol or denatured alcohol, which are poisonous when taken internally; stick with something from a liquor store. The authors also recommend 101 proof peppermint Schnapps. This high proof alcohol will easily dissolve the cannabinoids in the oil on the buds. Soaking an ounce of high quality bud in a pint of 101 proof peppermint Schnapps will produce a strong (let's repeat that: STRONG) elixir. If you like, a small amount of this can be put in a nice herbal tea to dilute the taste of the alcohol. The peppermint flavor of the Schnapps covers up any unpleasant flavors of the plant.

As always, the resulting tonic will be more potent if the grass is preheated so as to decarboxylate the THCA. This typically adds a slightly burned taste to the grass. Some people prefer the taste of fresh, green non-decarboxylated buds. They may also prefer the milder, less psychoactive effect resulting from a high ratio of THCA to active THC. It's conceivable that some people derive unique medical benefits from the THCA.

Be careful to measure the amount of marijuana you add so that the dose per unit of alcohol can be calculated. For instance, a fifth of alcohol is equal to 26 ounces. An ounce of marijuana is equal to 28 grams. Slightly less than one ounce of marijuana soaked in one fifth of alcohol would make 26 one-gram-per-ounce servings. If the amount of marijuana were doubled, a one-gram dose would be contained in one-half ounce of liquor.

Whole leaves can be added to the alcohol and are just as effective as ground marijuana, though their bulkiness makes them hard to stuff into a narrow-necked bottle. The alcohol can always be poured into a wide-necked jar for processing. This way, more leaf can be processed too. Once the processing is complete, the leaf is easily removed from the alcohol. Be sure to press the alcohol from the leaf before you discard it. (If the leaf is placed in a narrow-necked bottle, it doesn't have to be removed and can be discarded with the empty bottle.)

Some people prefer to add ground marijuana to the alcohol. It's less messy, easier to handle, and much less bulky, so a greater concentration is possible. To remove the remains, just pour the mixture out through a coffee filter. Alternatively, add the whole leaves to alcohol and run them through a blender, then filter.

Glycerin-based Cannabis Tincture

Even very small amounts of alcohol may be inappropriate for some patients. In that case, substitute vegetable glycerin (available at most large drug stores) for alcohol to make an effective tincture. Use the glycerin tincture just as you would one made with alcohol:

> 64 grams (approximately 2¼ ounces) of marijuana leaf
> 1 pint of vegetable glycerin

As with the alcohol tincture, the leaf may be ground and/or soaked in water before adding it to the glycerin. Mix the leaf and the glycerin in a suitable jar. Mint, lavender, or other herbs can be added at this stage as flavorings, if desired. The glycerin imparts a sweet, honey-like taste to the tincture.

Let the glycerin and leaf mixture stand in a dark place for 60 days. Shake the jar for about 3 minutes each day to ensure thorough mixing. After 60 full days, use a French press or coffee filter to strain the leaf out of the tincture. Heat the strained tincture to 212 degrees F (100° C) for 90 minutes or 390° F (200° C) for five minutes to decarboxylate the THC and activate the tincture. Use a candy thermometer to measure the temperature; glycerin boils at 554° F (290° C).

Marijuana Cooking Oil

THC-containing oil is also easy to make. Just add the marijuana to any vegetable oil and heat it to extract and decarboxylate the THCA. The oil prepared by this method can be used in any recipe that calls for vegetable oil – even salad dressings.

> 1 pint olive oil
> 64 grams dry weight (approx. 2¼ oz.) washed, ground leaf

Do not heat the oil directly on a stovetop. The heat is too high and you will end up with fried grass. Instead, place the oil and leaf flour in a crockpot or similar slow cooker. Cover the cooker and heat the marijuana-oil mixture on high for 1 hour, then on low for 2-3 hours more, stirring occasionally. Allow to cool, then strain the mixture through a cheesecloth or fine-mesh tea strainer. Press the oily leaf in the strainer with a spoon to squeeze the remaining oil out. Each half-tablespoon of oil will contain a one-gram portion.

Alternatively, you can leave the leaf in the oil. Before using, shake or stir the oil to mix the marijuana throughout, then measure out the amount desired.

Marijuana Butter (or Margarine)

Marijuana butter takes a little more effort, but is still quite easy to make.

2 sticks butter (8 oz.)

16 ounces water

32 grams leaf

Heat the water and butter together in a pot. Add the marijuana and stir occasionally. Keep simmering for about a half hour. Then remove the leaf from the mixture. Put the pot in the refrigerator. The butter will solidify at the top of the water. Discard the water. The marijuana butter is now ready to use in your favorite recipe, or just as a spread on some bread. One half tablespoon of butter equals a one-gram portion.

Dave's Famous Cookies, formerly sold at the S.F. Cannabis Buyers' Club, were made using a simple technique. Dave prepared the dried marijuana by removing all stems, then powdered it using a blender. Then he strained it to remove any leaf stems. He added this to a mixture of butter and oil, heated it until it simmered, then added the oil with the marijuana to an almond cookie batter with chocolate chips.

We once tasted a truly delicious marijuana cake prepared by

an acquaintance. He confided his secret: shortbread mix and marijuana rum. Certainly marijuana can be added to any cake or cookie mix, or you can use your own favorite recipe. You can use an alcohol or butter extract to add THC or, in some cases, add the marijuana directly to the mix.

Spicy corn bread was served at a recent dinner given by some S.F. Buyers' Club members. The recipe was taken right from the box, except that powdered marijuana was added. Each square contained about 1/8 gram of leaf. The hosts realized that guests would be eating more than one piece, so they kept the concentration low.

Many marijuana recipes use chocolate and coffee. These two flavors mask the marijuana taste well. Probably the best-known recipe is the famous "marijuana brownie" first popularized in Alice B. Toklas's 1930s cookbook.

The following recipes, which have been developed by medical users, are delicious with or without the marijuana.

BEVERAGES
Lhassi (One serving)

> 1 cup yogurt
> 1 cup crushed ice
> Sugar, honey, or other sweetening to taste
> Tiny pinch powdered cardamom (optional)
> Tiny pinch powdered cloves (optional)
> Few drops rosewater (optional)
> 1 portion marijuana butter or oil

Place all ingredients in a blender. Blend on the high setting until all the ice is thoroughly mixed in. Very refreshing on a hot day.

Marijuana Liqueur

    1 pint liqueur (16 ounces)

    8 grams (dry weight) whole presoaked leaf

Place the marijuana in a covered jar with the liqueur. Store in a cool, dark place until you remember it, but for at least three days. Pour and serve. You may wish to remove the leaves for aesthetic reasons. Each ounce of liqueur is one half-gram serving.

Marijuana Milk

Heat a glass of milk or soymilk over a low flame on the stove or in a microwave oven. When it is warm, add one portion or more of water-treated marijuana. Keep the mixture warm, just below simmering, for half an hour. Strain the mix and discard the leaf. This milk can be used for cooking or drinking, or mixed with cereal.

DESSERTS
The Ultimate Gourmet Brownie

    6 oz. high-quality bittersweet chocolate

    1/2 cup marijuana butter

    4 tbsp chocolate syrup

    2 tbsp unsweetened cocoa

    1 tsp almond extract

    4 egg whites, beaten fluffy

    3/4 cup sugar

    1/8 tsp salt

    1/2 cup flour

    1 tsp baking powder

Melt chocolate, chocolate syrup, and cocoa over low heat, stirring constantly. Remove from the heat and stir in butter, oil, and egg whites. Mix thoroughly. Add salt, flour, sugar, and baking powder and blend completely. Pour into an 8" square baking pan and place in a preheated 350° F (177° C) oven for 30 minutes.

Of course, you can add nuts, coconut, or chocolate chips to the mix before you bake it. This makes sixteen 2" square brownies. Each square contains 1 gram of marijuana

Tom's Carrot Cake

We discovered this great recipe for carrot cake in Tom Flowers' book, *Marijuana Herbal Cookbook*. He kindly allowed us to reprint it here.

    6 oz. butter
    1/4-1/2 oz. marijuana leaf
    1 cup finely grated carrot
    3/4 cup brown sugar
    3/4 cup milk
    2 large eggs
    1/2 cup shredded coconut
    1 tsp grated orange peel
    1 tsp ginger
    1 3/4 cup flour
    1 tbsp baking powder

Beat softened butter and marijuana leaf. Add the carrot, sugar, milk, eggs, coconut, orange peel, and ginger. When this is thoroughly mixed, sift in flour and baking powder.

When everything is thoroughly mixed, pour the batter into an 8" square baking pan. Bake for 45 minutes at 325° F (163° C). This makes 16 slices.

Chocolate Pudding

You can prepare commercial chocolate pudding from a package (if you don't mind the list of ingredients in it!). This is how to do it:

> 1 package chocolate pudding mix
> 4 portions marijuana butter, oil, milk, alcohol, or ground leaf

Prepare the pudding as directed. Add marijuana or extract to the mix when you add the milk or soymilk. For good portion control, pour into serving dishes while the pudding is still warm.

You can also make pudding for yourself. Here's another great recipe from Tom Flower's Marijuana Herbal Cookbook.

Mile High Chocolate Pudding

Mix together:

> 1/4 cup water
> 3 tbsp cornstarch

Set aside. Whisk together in a saucepan:

> 1 egg (optional)
> 2 cups milk or soymilk
> 1 to 4 teaspoons of marijuana leaf flour or 0.5 to 2 grams of marijuana bud flour
> 3 tbsp sugar
> 6 tbsp cocoa

Heat on low, stirring occasionally to keep it from sticking to the bottom of the pan. Just before the mix boils, stir the cornstarch and water and pour the blend into the mixture, stirring quickly until the mixture thickens. Serve hot or cold. Makes 4 ½ cup servings.

SAUCES
Tomato Sauce from a Jar

Marijuana can be simply prepared with a commercial tomato sauce. Take a half jar of sauce and add about 2 grams of nice-quality leaf in a pouch made of nylon netting, which can be bought at a home brew store. Push this into the tomato sauce (which should contain oil) and heat the mix in the microwave until boiling. Let the mix sit for about an hour, stirring about every 15 minutes. Then heat it up again, remove the pouch, and serve pasta for four.

Non-Food Ingestion Preparations—Capsules

Eating marijuana in food is a fine way of getting the medicine. However, it's not necessary to eat constantly to get relief. Clients of many buyers' clubs have found that marijuana capsules are a convenient way to take the herb.

Marijuana capsules are simple to make. First, at a health food store or drugstore, buy capsules of a size that is convenient for you to swallow. Then make a paste of one gram ground marijuana, a drop of lecithin, and just enough olive oil to make the paste on the dry side. Pre-heating the marijuana to decarboxylate the THC-acid can enhance the potency of the capsules. Stuff the bottom part of the capsule with the paste. At the San Francisco Buyers' Club, one gram of marijuana was stuffed into four capsules. This was convenient for the clients, who could use just a portion of the dose at a time.

Some stores and mail-order houses offer capsule stuffers. These devices hold the capsule bottoms in place for easy filling, then once they're filled allow you to tamp them all at once.

Chapter 8
Dealing with Drug Testing

Drug testing is one of the most troublesome problems confronting medical marijuana patients. Drug urine screening has become increasingly pervasive in the American workplace in recent years. It is also being used, with no good scientific justification, as a test for driving under the influence in certain states.

By far the most widely used and objectionable form of drug testing is urinalysis. Urine tests are uniquely over-sensitive to marijuana, traces of which are detectable for days or even weeks after last use, long after its effects have faded. This is far longer than the detection time for other, more dangerous drugs such as heroin, methamphetamine, or cocaine—not to mention alcohol, the most commonly abused drug of all, which is barely detectable in urine and rarely screened for at all in workplace drug programs.

Urine tests in no way detect whether one is actually under the influence of marijuana. That's because they don't actually measure THC, but rather non-psychoactive cannabinoid metabolites that are produced by the liver and linger in the system long after the effects of THC have passed away. In particular, urine tests detect a substance known as THC-COOH (11-nor-9-carboxy-THC), sometimes referred to as an acid, but not to be confused with the THC acid that is found in the plant and is a precursor to THC.

Although THC-COOH is not psychoactive, there is some evidence that it may have analgesic and anti-inflammatory properties [Burstein1]. THC-COOH rises steadily in the urine for the first few hours after smoking, then tails off over a period of days (or a period of weeks with regular users, in whom cannabinoids and metabolites accumulate in bodily fat over time, gradually releasing after cessation of use). It must be stressed that there is no correlation between urine THC-COOH levels and a current state of intoxication. The presence of THC-COOH and other metabolites indicates that substantial metabolic degradation has already taken place in the body.

For this reason, urine tests are incapable of distinguishing between occasional, weekend use and on-the-job use or impairment. This is why even the US Department of Justice admits that "a positive test result, even when confirmed ... does not indicate abuse or addiction, recency, frequency, amount of use, or impairment" [DOJ2]. Unfortunately, this has not stopped the widespread misuse of urine testing as a supposed test for drug abuse, much like the misuse of loyalty oaths and lie detectors in days gone by.

Frequent and infrequent marijuana users are similar in the way they metabolize THC, which leads to many misinterpretations. Another fact frequently overlooked is that most absorbed THC is eliminated in feces, with only about 33 percent being elimi-

---

1 Burstein S, "Therapeutic Potential of Ajulemic Acid (CT3)" in Grotenhermen & Russo, pp. 381-2.
2 US Department of Justice, Bureau of Justice Statistics. Drugs, Crime, and the Justice System (NCJ-133652). December 1992, p. 119.

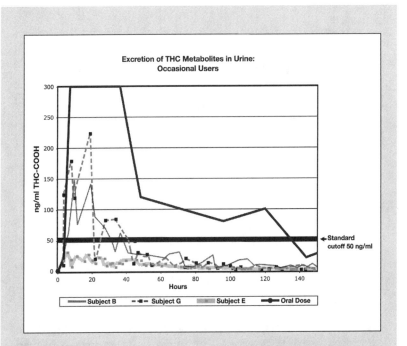

Figure 1. Excretion of THC Metabolites in Urine – Occasional Users

Urine testing profiles for occasional users (once a week or less) who are clean before taking marijuana. The standard cutoff for workplace drug tests is 50 ng.ml; confirmation tests are sensitive to 15 ng. Subjects B, G, E received identical doses of one joint. Typical users like (B) and (G) test positive for a day or two after smoking. Note that metabolite levels may seesaw above and below the cutoff. Urine remained negative at 50 ng for first 3.5 hours after dosing. Unusual subjects such as (E) may not test positive at all. (D) A strong oral dose of 20 mg produced positive drug test results for six days. In rare instances, detection times of two weeks may occur.

REFERENCE, FIGURE 1. Subjects B, G, E from M. Huestis, J. Mitchell and E. Cone, "Urinary Excretion Profiles of 11-Nor-9-Carboxy-Delta9-Tetrahydrocannabinol in Humans after Single Smoked Doses of Marijuana," Journal of Analytical Toxicology 20: 441-452 (1996). Oral dose from B. Law et al, "Forensic aspects of the metabolism and excretion of cannabinoids following oral ingestion of cannabis resin," J. Pharm. Pharamacol. 36:289-294 (1983).

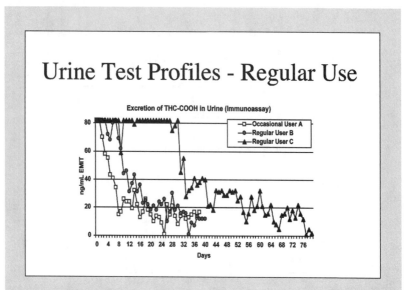

Figure 2: Urine Testing Profiles – Regular Use

In regular users, metabolite levels can build up to 1,000 ng or more, requiring weeks to clean out. On this graph, detection times ranged from a week to a month at the standard detection cutoff of 50 ng. Detection times of over 100 days have been reported.

REFERENCE, FIGURE 2 Graph courtesy of Franjo Grotenhermen, based on data in GM Ellis et al., "Excretion patterns of cannabinoid metabolites after last use in a group of chronic users." Clin Pharmacol Ther 38(5):572-578 (1985).

nated in the urine. Happily, drug testing companies have not had the stomach to promote excrement testing!

Blood Tests

Other kinds of tests can be used to detect marijuana. The most accurate of these is blood testing, which measures the actual presence of THC in the bloodstream. In general, blood testing is a much better, though imperfect, gauge of recent impairment, since it detects the presence of the psychoactive drug in the sys-

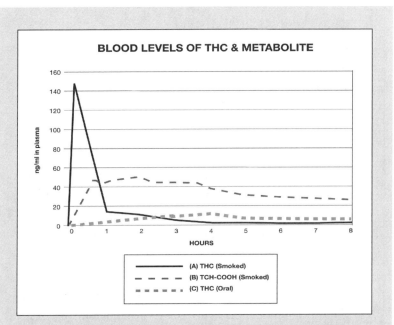

Figure 3: Blood Levels of THC and Metabolite

(A) THC peaks sharply in first few minutes after smoking then tails off to levels beneath 5-10 ng within a couple of hours. THC may remain at detectable levels of 2 ng/ml for 12 hours after a single use or up to a week in chronic users.

(B) Inactive metabolite THC-COOH lingers at higher levels in blood for three days or as long as a week in occasional users and weeks in regular users.

(C) When consumed orally, THC rises slowly to a low plateau of 3 to 11 ng. THC-COOH reaches similar levels as with smoked marijuana after a couple of hours (not shown).

REFERENCES, FIG. 3 (A-B) based on data from M. Huestis, J. Henningfield and E. Cone, "Blood Cannabinoids. I. Absorption of HTC and Formation of 11-OH-THC and THCCOOH During and After Smoking Marijuana," Journal of Analytic Toxicology, Vol. 16: 276-282 (1992). (C) based on data from B. Law et al, "Forensic aspects of the metabolism and excretion of cannabinoids following oral ingestion of cannabis resin," J. Pharm. Pharamacol. 36:289-294 (1983).

tem. Blood tests typically register positive for just a few hours after use. However, chronic users may show detectable levels of 1 or 2 nanograms per milliliter (ng/ml) for up to two days without being appreciably impaired. When smoking, THC levels peak sharply within the first 10 minutes, sometimes to levels above 100 ng/ml, then drop quickly to single digits, finally tailing off over the next few hours. When consumed orally, THC levels rise to a lower, broader plateau about an hour after consumption, continuing for 4-6 hours.

Blood tests are often used after accidents to determine whether the subject was under the influence of marijuana. Although less over-sensitive than urine tests, blood tests are not a perfect indicator of impairment. Accident studies have found that drivers who test positive at low levels of THC – typically below the threshold of 3.5 to 5 nanograms per milliliter in blood – are no more dangerous than drug-free drivers [Grotenhermen3]. On the other hand, levels above 3.5 to 5 nanograms of THC indicate likely impairment. Typically, levels above 5 nanograms persist only for the first hour or so after smoking, and levels in this range are more consistent with acute intoxication. However, as with many drugs, frequent users may not be functionally impaired by cannabinoid levels in this range.

In recent years, advocates of drug testing have pushed to mandate so-called "per se" standards for driving under the influence of cannabis, similar to the legal standard of 0.08% blood alcohol for drunken driving. The idea is to set a certain threshold above which it is automatically assumed that the driver is intoxicated. Although this seems like a sensible principle, it has been impossible to realize in practice, because scientific studies have failed to demonstrate a clear threshold for impairment for drugs other than alcohol.

However, this hasn't stopped some states and countries from

---

3 Grotenhermen F. et al, "Developing Science-Based Per Se Limits for Driving under the Influence of Cannabis (DUIC): Findings and Recommendations by an Expert Panel," Hürth, Germany: Nova-Institut (2005) http://www.canorml.org/healthfacts/DUICreport.2005.pdf ; summarized in "Developing Limits for Driving Under Cannabis" Addiction 102(12):1910-1917 (2007).

trying to legislate them anyhow. Some have even gone so far as to establish a zero-tolerance threshold for marijuana or metabolites, even though the evidence is clear that low levels of marijuana are compatible with safe driving. An international expert review panel recommended a per se standard of 3.5 to 5 milligrams per THC in blood based on scientific reviews of accident safety [Grotenhermen[4]]. However, even this limit is arbitrary, as some drivers can drive safely at higher levels. In one study, a subject with severe attention deficit/hyperactivity disorder could not pass a driving test while straight, but performed well under the influence of cannabis with a THC blood level of 71 ng/ml [Strohbeck-Kühner[5]]! No similar phenomenon is known to occur in connection with alcohol.

In addition to THC, blood tests can also detect the metabolites of marijuana. These include THC-COOH, the primary inactive metabolite, and 11-OH(hydroxy)-THC, the psychoactive metabolite that is produced when marijuana is ingested. THC-COOH stays in the body longer than THC, rising to significant levels an hour after smoking and tailing off over a few days. The presence of THC-COOH is not an indication of being under the influence.

The psychoactive metabolite, 11-OH-THC, does not occur in significant quantities when marijuana is inhaled. When ingested, the blood levels of 11-OH-THC tend to track those of THC, slowly rising to a broad plateau for 2-6 hours after use.

Some experts claim they can accurately estimate the time at which one has last used marijuana by analyzing the ratios of THC, 11-OH-THC and THC-COOH. However, this method has not been conclusively validated by controlled studies.

---

4 Ibid.
5 Strohbeck-Kühner et al, "Fahrtüchtigkeit trotz (wegen) THC" ["Driving ability despite (or because of) THC"], Archiv für Kriminologie 220:11-19 (2007).

Hair Tests

Hair testing can also be used to detect marijuana use. This method is especially obnoxious because it cannot measure current use, but only use that has occurred days, weeks or months in the past. Hair strand testing detects the presence of drug metabolites that have passively diffused from the blood stream to the base of the hair follicle. The drug residues are incorporated into the hair and remain detectable until it grows out or is cut. Hair tests are less sensitive to marijuana than cocaine and other drugs, and more likely to detect frequent than occasional use. A NIDA study of 38 marijuana users found that 85% of those who used daily tested positive in hair, compared to only 52% of those who used marijuana 1-5 times per week; altogether, 36% of subjects tested negative [Huestis[6]]. Although other studies have found that hair tests are more sensitive to dark than light hair, especially for cocaine, this study found no difference between Caucasians and African-Americans. Since the results of hair tests bear no relation to job performance, their use is unfairly discriminatory. However, this hasn't stopped them from being used by certain unscrupulous employers as well as by the criminal justice system.

A number of shampoos are hawked on the market, which claim to help marijuana smokers pass hair tests. These may be helpful in removing external drug residues, such as marijuana smoke particles that stick to the hair. However, they are less likely to eliminate drug metabolites that have been incorporated into the hair follicles. There is no scientific evidence that commercially sold hair-test shampoos are more reliable or effective in defeating hair tests. This would seem to be theoretically impossible anyway, as the metabolites are inside the structure of the hair shaft itself.

---

6 Huestis M, et al, "Cannabinoid concentrations in hair from documented cannabis users," Forensic Science International . 169.2-3:129-36 (2007).

Saliva Tests

Another kind of drug test currently under development is saliva testing. Saliva tests offer the major advantage of being less invasive of bodily privacy than urine or blood tests. They are now commonly used in obtaining DNA samples for forensic evidence. In principle, saliva testing should detect THC residues for a fairly limited time after use – a few hours – giving a good indication of recent usage. In practice, however, the technology has not yet achieved acceptable accuracy and reliability for wide-scale use. One study found that only one out of 18 known THC-positive subjects tested positive in saliva [Kintz[7]]. Another review of ten separate oral fluid, point-of-collection drug testing devices reported that the devices failed to detect various controlled substances, including THC and its inactive metabolite THC-COOH, at cutoff concentrations recommended by the manufacturers [Walsh[8]].

Dealing With Urine Tests

Ideally, if marijuana was handled like other, legal drugs, workers wouldn't be denied employment on the basis of positive urine test results for marijuana, especially if they were using it for medical reasons. Workers are generally allowed to test positive for drugs for which they have a legal medical prescription. When a worker tests positive for a drug, a medical review officer checks the results and determines whether there is a legitimate medical excuse for the positive rest. Thus, an MRO will excuse a positive test for opiates if the worker has presented a legal prescription for codeine or oxycodone.

---

7 Kintz P, et al, "Detection of cannabis use in drivers with the drugwipe device and by GC-MS after Intercept device collection," Journal of Analytical Toxicology 29.7:724-7 (2005).
8 Walsh JM, et al, "Evaluation of Ten Oral Fluid Point-of-Collection Drug-Testing Devices," Journal of Analytical Toxicology 31.1: 44-54 (2007).

The problem, of course, is that marijuana isn't legal under federal law, so most companies don't allow it. In those states where marijuana is legal, some employers do allow exemptions for legal medical patients. However, this is the exception, not the rule. Few nationwide corporations allow medical marijuana, and none allow it in jobs subject to federal drug testing regulations, such as the transportation industry.

If you are faced with an employment drug test, it is worth inquiring discreetly whether the company's policy allows for medical marijuana. If not, here are some alternatives to consider.

(1) **Get a Marinol® prescription before the test.** Because Marinol contains THC, it is indistinguishable from marijuana on standard urine tests. Since it is also an FDA approved prescription drug, it offers a legal, acceptable excuse for a positive urine test. In order to use this excuse, you will have to inform the employer beforehand that you are using Marinol on your pre-physical questionnaire, where you are instructed to list prescribed drugs. In principle, this should protect against a THC-positive drug test result. Beware, though: some employers may refuse to accept use of Marinol (or other legal drugs) by their workers on the grounds that it renders them unfit for the job. In principle, advanced drug testing technology can distinguish Marinol from marijuana by testing for naturally occurring cannabinoids not found in Marinol. However, such testing is very expensive and has been used in only a handful of extraordinary cases involving the criminal justice system. Perhaps the biggest problem with the Marinol excuse, aside from economic cost, is that physicians are reluctant to prescribe it outside its labeled indications for cancer and HIV.

(2) **Don't rely on excuses.** If you test positive for marijuana, it's no use trying to claim that the test is wrong. False positives due to lab errors, while possible, are rare and never an accept-

able excuse. In case of a disagreement, the company will accept the lab's story, not yours. The standard procedure for conducting urine tests is to first check the sample with an immunoassay screen (such as the EMIT test), then, if the results are positive, confirm them with the more accurate gas chromatograph mass spectrometer (GCMS). This virtually eliminates the chance of false positives in exchange for a relatively high rate of false negatives where drug use is not detected. Federal regulations require backup GCMS tests in government-mandated testing programs. However, these regulations don't cover most private employers or pre-employment testing programs, which may fail to employ proper testing and backup procedures. In such cases, there may be an appreciable risk of false positives.

Aside from Marinol, there are no legal drugs that can cause a positive urine test for marijuana. One partial exception is the acid-reflux drug Protonix®, whose FDA label bears a warning that false urine screens for marijuana are possible. However, this confusion can be eliminated by means of a GCMS back-up test.

The hemp food products sold in grocery stores contain minuscule amounts of cannabinoids, but can't cause positive drug tests even in heavy doses. At one time this was a problem, but it was fixed by the hemp industry, which strengthened standards so as to strictly limit the level of THC in industrial hemp to negligible levels.

Another unacceptable excuse for positive drug tests is passive smoking of marijuana. Studies have shown that only under extreme conditions can passive exposure to marijuana smoke produce a positive drug test in a non-smoker: for example, by being repeatedly locked in an unventilated closet with half a dozen heavy smokers for hours on end. The odds of detecting passive exposure are less unrealistic if the test has a sensitive cutoff like 20 ng/ml. A more likely source of accidental exposure is inadvertently eating a marijuana-tainted edible. Naïve guests have been known to eat the wrong brownie at a party and end up flunking a drug test.

(3) **Clean out before the test.** The surest way to pass a urine test is to be clean when you take it. Unfortunately, this isn't possible in every situation, especially in workplaces that impose random testing on short notice. However, if you're looking for a job and expect to take a pre-employment test, you should have plenty of time to clean out.

How much time is necessary to get marijuana out of your system? Unfortunately, there is no simple answer to this question. Drug test results are extremely capricious, depending not only on the last time you used marijuana, but also how much you used, your usage pattern in prior days, your size, metabolism and genetic makeup, the state of your bladder and kidneys, and other unknowable factors. As a rule of thumb, a single isolated use of marijuana will not be detected on standard drug screens beyond 2–4 days, and sometimes a single day (see Fig. 1). On occasion, however, one-time use may show up for 5–7 days, and even longer times have been reported anecdotally in exceptional cases. Daily users take longer to clear out due to the build-up of cannabinoid metabolites in their system (Fig 2). In general, two or three weeks are sufficient, with a month being almost certain to clear the body for most users. However, unusually heavy chronic users have been known to test positive for 4–8 weeks or more. Aside from abstinence, there are no proven techniques for cleaning out. Although many users embark on elaborate exercise, dieting, and flushing regimes, there's no evidence that any of these are effective, and some may even be harmful.

Even longer detection times are possible if employers use more sensitive detection limits. The standard sensitivity threshold required by the federal government's drug-free workplace regulations is 50 nanograms per milliliter of marijuana metabolite. Some employers use the more generous cutoff of 100 nanograms. Others use a strict standard of 20 nanograms.

If you're preparing for a drug test, you might want to test yourself first. Numerous home testing kits and services are available on the Internet. Be sure that the test you are using is at least as sensitive as that which you will have to submit to (usually 50 nanograms). Also, beware that urine levels of marijuana metabolite fluctuate, so it is possible to pass a test then fail it the next day without using any marijuana in between. Typically, metabolite levels build up in your system overnight so that your first urine in the morning tends to be dirtier.

A good strategy for improving your odds on a drug test is to drink lots of liquid immediately prior to the test so as to stimulate your urine flow and dilute the concentration of drugs in the sample below the detection threshold. Water alone works fine. A number of pricey detox drinks, herbal teas, and oral additives are on the market that purport to help pass drug tests, but it is unproven that any are more effective than water. There is no evidence that drinking over many days helps flush the system – the important thing is drinking a couple of hours before the test.

If you're desperate, you may boost your urine flow by taking a diuretic drug or "water pill." Diuretics are commonly prescribed for hypertension and other diseases. Milder non-prescription diuretics include coffee, cranberry juice, beer, and certain pills for premenstrual water retention. A number of diets and flushing regimes have been proposed on the theory that they help cleanse the system over a period of days or weeks. However, there is no evidence that any of them work. There are also a number of substances alleged to "mask" or "detoxify" urine samples if taken orally, among them golden seal, aspirin, zinc sulfate, and various commercial products. These claims have no scientific basis. The only proven technique is to drink lots of fluid shortly before the test.

In a study of urine dilution, researchers compared subjects using plain water, two herbal drinks – Goldenseal root and a commercial product called Naturally Klean Herbal Tea–and a prescription diuretic [Cone[9]]. Marijuana metabolite concentrations dropped rapidly for all subjects, with false negatives occurring 1.5 to 2 hours after ingestion of about 2 quarts of fluid. Metabolite levels returned to normal over a period of 8 to 10 hours.

Beware, however: urine dilution can only be taken so far. Labs can detect when urine becomes excessively dilute and watery by measuring a substance known as creatinine in the urine. If the lab determines that your sample is too diluted, they will reject it. In most cases, they will allow you to take a second test. Of course, this gives you more time to clean out, but only if you haven't made the mistake of toking up in the meantime. Certain commercial detox drinks contain supplements that purport to raise the level of creatinine in the urine, but scientific tests indicate that they are not effective [Ropero-Miller[10]]. Another popular detox ingredient is Vitamin B-2, which colors the urine yellow so as to make it appear less watery. It's conceivable that such additives may slightly raise the odds of passing a test. However, urine dilution is never infallible, especially for heavy, long-time users.

Tampering

The last and lowest resort for patients desperate to pass a test is to tamper with the sample. Ethical issues aside, this is a danger-

9 Cone E "In Vivo Adulteration: Excess Fluid Ingestion Causes False-Negative Marijuana and Cocaine Urine Test Results," Journal of Analytical Toxicology 22.6:460-73 (1998).
10 Ropero-Miller JD, et al, "Effect of oral creatine supplementation on random urine creatinine, pH, and specific gravity measurements," Clin Chem 46.2:295-7 (2000).

ous course since testers are on the lookout for cheats and certain to flunk them if they get caught. On the other hand, extreme measures may be justified in emergency situations when drug tests are unscrupulously sprung by surprise or without good cause, as in random drug testing programs.

Sample collection facilities are supposed to take measures to discourage sample tampering – for example, checking IDs, requiring subjects to empty their pockets before the test, and preventing access to water or soap that could be used to adulterate the sample. In high-security institutions, such as prisons, urination may even be observed. However, undercover tests by the U.S. General Accounting Office found that 22 out of 24 collection sites for the transportation industry did not comply with all of the security protocols required by the Department of Transportation [GAO11]. In 8 out of 8 cases, GAO investigators successfully tampered with the sample by substituting clean urine or adding adulterants.

The most foolproof method for foiling a drug test is to substitute clean urine. It's important to keep the sample at body temperature (90°–98.5°), since this is checked at the point of collection. If you can't find clean urine elsewhere, you can buy it from various companies that specialize in drug testing aids. Kits with synthetic clean urine and temperature-control dispensers are available through the Internet except in certain states that ban them by law, which include Arkansas, Illinois, Kentucky, New Jersey, North and South Carolina, and Oklahoma.

In desperate situations, it's possible to foil the tests by throwing a chemical adulterant into the sample. The problem is that any

---

11 GAO (General Accounting Office), "Undercover Tests Reveal Significant Vulnerabilities in DOT's Drug Testing Program," Testimony before the Subcommittee on Highways and Transit, Committee on Transportation and Infrastructure, House of Representatives, Nov. 1, 2007.

adulterant can be detected by appropriate lab tests. However, for economic reasons, labs don't typically perform complete security tests on all samples. A number of everyday household products are known to produce false negatives on urine screens for marijuana, among them bleach, vinegar, ascorbic acid, salt, soap, and eye drops. Most of these are easily detectable by integrity tests that are routinely conducted by many labs, which include tests of acidity (PH) and density (specific gravity).

Eye drops are the one common adulterant most likely to elude routine integrity tests [Dasgupta[12]]. A number of more sophisticated urine test adulterants are commercially sold in states that allow them, among them Stealth® (containing peroxidase and peroxide), Klear® (nitrite), Instant Clean® (glutaraldehyde) and Urine Luck® (pyridinium chlorochromate or PCC). The drug testing industry is well aware of these products and constantly developing new methods for detecting them. This has led to a kind of arms race between testers and the drug test evasion industry. Despite the risks involved, companies selling drug-testing aids report fairly high success rates with adulterants and detox drinks. In the GAO investigation, labs failed to detect adulterants in 4 out of 4 samples submitted.

Avoiding On-Cause Testing

Drug tests are often required in the event of accidents on the job, driving violations, suspected drug violations, etc. Such tests are described as "on-cause" testing, although they often detect drug use that occurred long ago and is therefore irrelevant to the incident in question. In some instances, subjects of on-cause testing are allowed to determine the kind of drug test they are given. If

---

12 Dasgupta A, "The Effects of Adulterants and Selected Ingested Compounds on Drugs-of-Abuse Testing in Urine," American Journal of Clinical Pathology 128:491-503 (2007).

you are a marijuana user but not actually under the influence of marijuana at the time, your best course is to ask for a blood test. This is because blood tests usually register positive for THC for only a couple of hours after use, while urine tests, which detect metabolites, register positive for days. On the other hand, if you have used marijuana recently, particularly in the last couple of hours, you may do better to go with a urine test. Even though you're likely to test positive, you will at least be able to argue that you weren't under the influence at the time. This won't be possible if they test your blood and find THC in it. Also, it can take over two hours for smoked marijuana to show up in urine, so you may actually pass if you just lit up a few minutes ago and haven't smoked much previously. In contrast, blood THC levels are highest in the first few minutes after smoking.

A number of states have passed zero-tolerance laws making it illegal to drive with any detectable amount of marijuana in your system. Zero-tolerance states include Arizona, Georgia, Illinois, Indiana, Iowa, Michigan, Ohio, Rhode Island, Utah and Wisconsin, plus numerous European countries. If you are stopped by the police in such a state and required to take a drug test, you are at risk of imprisonment and losing your license. The best way to prevent this is to avoid accidents and traffic violations in the first place.

Not uncommonly, police investigate minor traffic violators for driving under the influence. This is especially likely if you are driving erratically, or the police smell marijuana in your car. Usually, it is difficult and time-consuming for the police to conduct a drug test. In the case of blood tests, they may have to take you to the station to a nurse. Therefore, police will typically screen you for signs of driving under the influence before deciding to have you tested.

The most common procedure is to examine your performance on a roadside field sobriety test. Three particular tests have been scientifically validated as indicators of driving under the influence. If you pass them, you have a better chance of avoiding arrest for DUI.

(1) Horizontal and Vertical gaze nystagmus. In this test, you are asked to hold your head steady and follow with your eyes as the policeman moves his finger slowly back and forth before you. If your eye movements are jerky (a phenomenon known as nystagmus), or you jerk your head, it's an indicator of impairment. Unfortunately, it's impossible to test yourself for nystagmus, though a friend might help you do so, since it takes no special medical training. In any case, this test is more sensitive to alcohol than marijuana.

(2) Walk and Turn. In this test (also known as tandem walking), you are required to walk nine steps heel-to-toe in a straight line, turn around, and walk nine steps back. If you stray from the line, lose your balance, or fail to follow instructions carefully, you're considered impaired. You can improve your performance on this test by simply practicing at home, as is true of most other motor performance tests.

(3) One Leg Standing. In this test, you must stand on one leg for 30 seconds with the other leg stretched straight in front of you six inches off the ground. If you lose your balance, hop, or put your foot to the ground, it's a sign of impairment. This is the best and most sensitive test of marijuana impairment. It is also easy to perform on yourself.

A good way to figure out whether you're fit to drive is to see whether you can perform the one-leg standing test. Some people have difficulty performing it even when stone cold sober. Such people are unfortunately vulnerable to arrest for DUI. Most people have no trouble with the one-leg standing test unless they are stoned or drunk. If you are one of them, avoid driving when you can't perform the test.

Another good test of impairment is your own subjective state of mind. If you find yourself unable to concentrate, losing track of what you're talking about, or forgetting where you are on the road, you're too stoned to drive. One simple test of your ability to concentrate is to count backwards from 100 in serial "3s" or "7s"—i.e. 100-97-94-91-88-85, etc. or 100-93-86-79-72, etc. Of course, some people can do this much better than others, but most everyone can tell the difference between doing so straight or stoned.

A final word of caution: Statistically, driving an automobile is the most dangerous task any person will do in their lifetime, barring some notable exceptions such as climbing Mount Everest. During the Vietnam War, more American citizens were killed on our own highways than were killed as soldiers in the jungles of Vietnam. We leave you with that to contemplate.

Chapter 9
Choosing a Variety

Marijuana comes in many varieties. Dispensaries in California often offer 30 to 40 kinds, with colorful names such as Skunk, Purple, Kush, Afghan, Northern Lights, etc. Consumers should beware of taking these names too seriously, since there are no established procedures for identifying specific varieties and no quality control labs to check their identity. DEA restrictions on research prevent U.S. labs from testing samples from "illicit" sources in the medical cannabis market. Consumers therefore have no assurance that what is sold as "Indica Kush" in one place bears any resemblance to the "Indica Kush" sold elsewhere.

Nevertheless, there is usually a consistency among varieties in states where medical marijuana is available. So varieties labeled "Afgooey" at separate dispensaries are likely to be similar. At the better dispensaries, sales personnel are knowledgeable about their product and able to guide clients to an appropriate variety.

Indica and Sativa

Marijuana is usually divided into two broad categories: indicas and sativas. These two broad groups are often hybridized and referred to as sativa-indica or indica-sativa hybrids depending on the dominance of either type. Originally, the names sativa and indica designated two different naturalized species or landraces with distinct growing patterns from different parts of the world. These landraces have now been so interbred that the basis for the original distinction has become highly dubious. The distinction is further confused by the fact that there remains no scientifically agreed-upon definition for sativa or indica, nor any definitive analysis of their respective biochemical, pharmaceutical and genetic properties.

Nevertheless, there has emerged a popular consumer folklore about typical differences between indica and sativa varieties. Following this tradition, the authors offer the following impressionistic, anecdotal account of varietal differences based on visual appearance, odor, taste, and the personal experience of ourselves and others.

Sativas have fruity, floral and sweet aromas. They are said to be focusing, energizing and inspirational. This characteristic can be used to distance the mind from pain, and can be useful in conjunction with other activities such as internal imagery, breathing exercises, or artistic expression.

Indicas have a dry, acrid, even skunk-like odor. They are said to be relaxing, sleep-inducing, anti-nauseant, and relieving of stress and pain. The sedative effects are used to treat chronic pain, often in conjunction with a hot bath, massage or sauna. Patients report that they work synergistically with opiates and pain relievers. In contrast to sativas, indicas tend to be body-oriented and "stony."

These distinctions should not be taken too literally, since varieties can possess a mixture of characteristics. The differences probably had more meaning when marijuana growers were acquiring landraces. They have come to be blurred as plants have been bred and rebred, hybridized and then hybridized again with new introductions from all over the world.

In his book *The Botany of Desire*, Michael Pollan showed that prohibition has helped marijuana adapt to new environments such as the great indoors. Since marijuana gardeners don't have access to seeds as easily as flower and vegetable gardeners, they have reverted to home breeding. This may have made marijuana the plant with the largest breeding program, with test plots in countless closets and gardens as well as commercial establishments. The result of all of this is very mixed up strains. None of them are usually identifiable by landrace. Instead they are given fanciful or sometimes descriptive names.

TERPENES

For years researchers thought that different ratios of cannabinoids created marijuana's varying effects. However, studies of modern marijuana varieties show that most varieties contain large amounts of THC but hardly any of the other cannabinoids. This led researchers to take a second look at terpenes, the odor molecules found in plant essential oils.

Almost all plant odors, from perfumy flowers to herbs and spices, are composed of plant terpenes. Plants produce terpenes for several reasons: to attract pollinators, to attract predators of herbivores, and to repel or kill predators. Spices and herbs derive their characteristic odors from the essential oils they produce. Each plant's oil is a combination of different terpenes. Many terpenes are found in oils of different plants. For instance, limonene, which lends citrus its characteristic odor, is also found in spices such as rosemary, juniper, peppermint and marijuana.

Plant essential oils, each of which contains its own combination of terpenes, are used in aromatherapy because the terpenes affect our mood and brain function.

Scientists now think that different combinations of terpenes can account for the various medical benefits and mood alterations in different varieties of marijuana.

Just as rose varieties have different odors, marijuana varieties have unique odors ranging from sweet to skunky, from floral to acrid. Each of these odors indicates combinations of terpenes. Some of them, such as the various analogs of limonene, are familiar. The limonenes carry citrus odors such as orange, tangerine, lemon and grapefruit. Limonene is thought to enhance alertness and focused attention, and also has fungicidal properties.

Since the terpenes affect the marijuana experience, by learning to recognize some of the odors you can anticipate how a particular marijuana will affect you. Odor is your clue about the type of medicinal qualities. Marijuana varieties with similar odors will usually provide the same kind of relief.

Here are some of the other terpenes that are found in cannabis:

Myrcene

Myrcebe is the most prevalent terpene found in marijuana. Its odor is described as citrus, clove-like, earthy, fruity, green-vege-tative and mango. The differences in odor are the result of slight differences in the makeup of the molecule. Notice that all of these odors are used to describe marijuana. Myrcene is a potent analgesic, anti-inflammatory and antibiotic. It blocks the effects of the pro-mutagens implicated as carcinogens such as aflatoxin B. It is found in small amounts in many essential oils associated with anti-depressive and uplifting behavior.

Myrcene is probably a synergist of THC: a combination of the two molecules creates a stronger experience than THC alone. Myrcene probably affects the permeability of the cell membrane, allowing more THC to reach the brain.

Beta-caryophyllene

Beta-caryophyllene smells and tastes peppery, with hints of clove and camphor. It is a major component of oils of clove and black pepper. It has analgesic qualities, but doesn't have a mental effect. A recent study by Swiss researchers found that beta-caryophyllene binds to the CB-2 receptor and has anti-inflammatory effects in mice [Gertsch et al.[1]]. Beta-caryophyllene is therefore a kind of non-psychoactive cannabinoid analog.

Pinene

Pinene has a piney odor and is a major component of turpentine. It is found in pine trees as well as rosemary, sage and eucalyptus. It is thought to help memory by crossing the blood-brain barrier and inhibiting the activity of the chemical that destroys an information transfer molecule. As a result this molecule has a longer time to work before it is inactivated, resulting in better memory. It also increases focus, self-satisfaction and memory. The skunky odors of some marijuana varieties are created in large part by analogs of this terpene, which are indications of its presence.

1   Jürg Gertsch, Marco Leonti, Stefan Raduner, Ildiko Racz, Jian-Zhong Chen, Xiang-Qun Xie, Karl-Heinz Altmann, Meliha Karsak, and Andreas Zimmer. *Beta-caryophyllene is a dietary cannabinoid.* PNAS 2008 105:9099-9104; published ahead of print June 23, 2008, doi:10.1073/pnas.0803601105

Terpenol

Terpenol smells floral, with hints of lilac and orange blossom. Terpenol causes drowsiness, and a desire to rest. It is often found in cannabis in conjunction with pinene, which masks its odor. This is what causes some Afghan varieties to have such a sedative affect. It is useful for sleep problems, as well as being a general sedative.

Borneol

Borneol smells like menthol or camphor. It is considered calming in Chinese medicine and helps people relax.

Linalool

Linalool has a floral scent reminiscent of spring flowers such as lily of the valley, but with spicy overtones. It is a component of lavender oil. It is being tested for use on some cancers [Ravizza et al. [2]][Cherng et al.[3]][Russin et al.[4]]. It causes severe sedation when inhaled. Patients looking for help sleeping should seek a floral-sweet variety. For patients seeking a separation from body discomforts, some sativa varieties transport you to a different mental state that can range from focused to distracted, ultimately helping you to become less aware of the pain and discomfort. They often have a citrus or fruity odor. If you wish to remain conscious, beware of linalool's floral sweet undertones sub-

---

2 Ravizza R, Gariboldi MB, Molteni R, Monti E. *Linalool, a plant-derived monoterpene alcohol, reverses doxorubicin resistance in human breast adenocarcinoma cells.* Oncol Rep. 2008 Sep;20(3):625-30. PMID: 18695915 [PubMed - in process]

3 Cherng JM, Shieh DE, Chiang W, Chang MY, Chiang LC. *Chemopreventive effects of minor dietary constituents in common foods on human cancer cells.* Biosci Biotechnol Biochem. 2007 Jun;71(6):1500-4. PMID: 17587681 [PubMed - indexed for MEDLINE]

4 Russin WA, Hoesly JD, Elson CE, Tanner MA, Gould MN. *Inhibition of rat mammary carcinogenesis by monoterpenoids.* Carcinogenesis. 1989 Nov;10(11):2161-4. PMID: 2509095 [PubMed - indexed for MEDLINE]

tly hidden under the limonene-citrus odors. The linalool component overtakes the conscious space and puts you to sleep.

Pulgone

Pulgone has a minty-camphor odor and flavor used by candy makers. It is thought to slow the destruction of memory transfer proteins so memory is improved. It also helps keep you alert and may counteract the terpenol and linalool to some extent.

HOW TO SELECT A MARIJUANA VARIETY TO MATCH A PATIENT'S NEEDS

Once you have an idea of what kind of marijuana will meet your medical needs you should be able to select varieties that will provide the desired effects. If you are cultivating for yourself, you will also need to all consider what will do well in your garden. Some of the factors to consider when choosing a variety are whether it is an indoor or outdoor plant, the size and growing habits of the variety, its temperature preferences and light needs, and any other special requirements.

For purposes of illustration, the authors along with Rick Pfrommer of Harborside Health Center in Oakland, California, have sampled four varieties from a California dispensary, and analyzed them as examples of how a patient might judge them. The varieties are Grand Daddy Purple, OG Kush, Purple Kush, and Sour Diesel.

Grand Daddy Purple

Grand Daddy Purple is described by the dispensary as "The King of the Purps." This is the strain that many of the other purps were bred from. It is the ultimate calmative, sedative medicine and often used for pain relief. It is also indicated for treating insomnia, appetite stimulation, and spasticity.

In the *Big Book of Buds*, Grand Daddy Purple is described as having a subtle grape aroma and sweet grape taste. "Her buzz is surprisingly alert and energetic rather than sedating." Elsewhere, it is described as sweet and perfumey with a pungent bottom end [King[5]]. The high is strong and felt mostly in the body.

The tested sample was analyzed at 18% THC. It had an acrid odor with a faint synthetic grape taste similar to grape soda. We surmised that it contained significant amounts of pinene, limonene, borneol and contained moderate levels of myrcene and terpenol. The feeling was very pleasant, relaxed and clearheaded, but none of us felt high.

OG Kush

The dispensary provides this description of OG Kush:

> "The first shock wave hits hard. It doesn't take long to realize that you're already feeling its effects from just one or two hits. A few puffs and the effects are long lasting and intense, but beware that the recovery period is prolonged. This bud is more of a late night adventure than a midday smoke break....It is a good strain for treating social anxiety, stress, depression and for appetite stimulation."

The sample we tested had 34% THC. It had a musky odor, almost like smelly feet and earthy. In addition it had floral tones, and cut lawn and sage odors. We surmised that it contained large

5 King, J., *Cannabible* (Berkeley, Ten Speed Press, 2001).

amounts of myrcene, limonene, pinene, borneol and moderate amounts of linalool and pulgone.

The high was friendly, mind opening and meditative. It took us to "new places."

Purple Kush

Purple Kush is described by the dispensary as:

> "Its pain relieving effects are immediate. It's good for anxiety, depression, chronic pain, insomnia, stress and stomach disorders. The Kush high is a deep stone.

> "Its deep body stone delivers treatment for chronic pain, depression, insomnia, stress and stomach disorders.

> "The buds have a soft pine bouquet and a sweet, grapey taste on an earthy foundation. It has an indica taste."

The sample we tested had 29% THC. It smelled like over-ripe tropical fruit: guava, with overtones of anise. We surmised that it contained large quantities of myrcene and caryophyllene as well as pulgone and borneol.

The high was "generic," it had no character. We felt it was sort of neutral.

Sour Diesel

Sour Diesel is described by the dispensary as:

> "The buzz is a heady, thought-provoking sativa that takes the rider on a wandering trip with an element of body to it. Good for relaxing on the couch, yet does not restrict daytime functionality.

"It is recommended for MS/neuropathic pain, incontinence, focus/ADD and social anxiety.

"It has a distinct odor of grapefruit and other citrus."

The sample we tested had 17% THC. It smelled like sour grapefruit, a little bit of Christmas tree, and had a slight floral odor. We surmised it had high levels of limonene and moderate amounts of myrcene and pinene.

The effect was "psychedelic like 60's pot," functional—not crippling, mood elevating, with clarity.

Chapter 10
Obtaining Medical Marijuana

As of this writing, marijuana remains completely illegal under federal law. As a Schedule 1 drug under the U.S. Controlled Substances Act, it is regarded as having high abuse potential and no medical use. Its possession, sale, manufacture, transportation and distribution for any purpose are against federal law.

Significantly, however, a growing number of states have laws permitting medical use of marijuana (as of this writing, they number 12: Alaska, California, Colorado, Hawaii, Maine, Montana, Nevada, New Mexico, Oregon, Rhode Island, Vermont and Washington). Typically these laws exempt patients from criminal charges for personal possession and/or cultivation of small amounts if they have a doctor's recommendation.

Because the overwhelming majority of small-scale drug offenses are prosecuted under state law, this means that patients in medical marijuana states are generally safe from arrest provided they follow local rules. Exceptions involve violations on federal property, at immigration or customs checkpoints, and in federally sponsored housing and employment.

Although it would seem that the federal government has no right to deny Americans access to medicine, the Supreme Court has ruled otherwise. In *Gonzalez v. Raich* it determined that Congress may prohibit personal possession and cultivation of marijuana even by patients whose lives depend on it as part of its assumed powers to regulate interstate commerce. Despite the Raich decision, the federal government has avoided pursuing individual patients, instead focusing its enforcement efforts on high-profile suppliers and dispensaries.

The federal ban on marijuana has effectively prevented the establishment of fully legal commercial producers and distributors of pharmaceutical cannabis. Most states have been reluctant to allow distribution of medical cannabis in the presence of the federal ban. A notable exception has been in California, where many localities have allowed the establishment of medical cannabis dispensaries or "buyers' clubs." Despite scores of federal raids and prosecutions, the number of dispensaries in California has grown from a handful in 1996 to over 300 in 2007. A handful of dispensaries have begun to crop up elsewhere, in such places as Colorado, Washington, and Canada. New Mexico, the newest medical marijuana state as of this writing, is in the process of developing regulations for licensed producers, which could conceivably lead to either a state or private-run medical marijuana distribution system.

Prescription availability through licensed pharmacies remains completely blocked, since pharmacies are subject to extensive federal FDA and DEA drug regulations. As a result, U.S. patients must rely on home cultivation or alternative channels to obtain their medicine.

A few foreign countries have established legal suppliers of medical cannabis. In the Netherlands, the Dutch Office for Medicinal Cannabis has licensed a farm to provide cannabis for prescription in pharmacies. Its products, known as Bedrocan and Bedrobinol, are twice as expensive as the marijuana and hashish that are sold over the counter in Dutch coffee shops. The increased cost is due to careful quality control procedures that prevent contamination from mold, bacteria, pesticides, etc. Though Dutch patients can have their Bedrocan prescriptions paid for by the national health system, most seem happy to simply patronize the coffee shops. As a result, the demand for Dutch medical cannabis has been disappointing.

In Canada, unlike in the U.S., the nation's highest court ruled that the ban on medical marijuana was unconstitutional and ordered the government to provide legal access to medical marijuana. The government responded by establishing a complicated and bureaucratic patient registration program run by Health Canada. Patients must fill out a detailed set of application forms with help from their doctor. For conditions not on the government's list of approved indications (MS, spinal cord disease or injury, cancer, AIDS/HIV, severe arthritis and epilepsy), patients must get the approval of two doctors and demonstrate that other, conventional medications have failed. Approved patients have the choice of applying for permission to grow their own, or else purchasing medicine from a government-approved contractor, Prairie Plant Systems, which operates a garden in an abandoned mine in Flin Flon, Manitoba.

Canadian patients have complained in vain about the poor quality and high cost of the government's cannabis, Health Canada's onerous and complicated regulations, and a lack of cooperation by Canadian doctors. As a result, most Canadian patients currently get their medicine from friends or from the numerous non-legal "compassion clubs" that have sprung up to meet demand.

In Israel, a Tel Aviv clinic has quietly begun providing medical marijuana with the approval of the state Health Ministry. The medicine is supplied free of charge to patients with AIDS, cancer or Crohn's disease. The clinic produces its own, high quality marijuana at a secure indoor garden tended by an experienced medical grower.

In the U.S., the 12 states that have adopted medical marijuana laws typically make it legal for patients to possess and cultivate for personal medical use provided that they have a doctor's recommendation. They also allow patients to designate primary caregivers to help cultivate or obtain their medicine for them.

Austria has also moved to establish a national medical cannabis program.

Although state laws do not protect against federal laws on marijuana, in practice they provide protection for patients with small, personal use home gardens, since the federal government rarely concerns itself with small-scale growers unless they are on federal property.

Physician Recommendations

The first essential step in qualifying as a legal patient is to obtain a physician's recommendation (sometimes referred to as an approval or certification). A recommendation consists of a physician's written statement that marijuana would be medically beneficial for the patient's condition. Legally, recommendations differ from prescriptions, which are legally defined to mean a written order to a licensed pharmacist to supply the drug. Since marijuana is not available in licensed pharmacies, and prescription drugs are subject to extensive federal regulation, prescriptions for marijuana are impossible. (This effectively invalidates a medical marijuana law passed by Arizona voters in 1996, Proposition 200, which was ineptly worded so as to require patients seeking marijuana to obtain two "prescriptions." As a result, Arizona's law has been a dead letter).

In contrast, physicians may legally "recommend" marijuana as they please, according to a decision by the Ninth Circuit Court of Appeals, *Conant v. Walters* (2002). In its ruling, the Ninth Circuit found that the right of physicians to recommend drugs was protected under the First Amendment. The decision is binding on all federal courts in the Ninth Circuit, which includes the West Coast. The Supreme Court effectively conceded its validity by refusing to hear an appeal. Under the Conant decision, physicians who recommend marijuana are protected from federal persecution so long as they do not get involved in its actual distribution, production or acquisition. Thousands of physicians are now recommending marijuana to their patients under state medical marijuana laws, and so far not one has been punished by the federal government for doing so.

Nonetheless, many physicians still remain reluctant to recommend marijuana. Some do so wrongly out of misplaced concern about the threat of federal arrest. Others are simply ill-informed about marijuana's benefits. Still others see marijuana as lying outside the mainstream of medicine because of its federal illegality and lack of FDA approval. As we noted in Chapter 1, many professional medical associations have gone on record in support of medical marijuana. Unfortunately, some medical societies still have not, among them the American (and Canadian) Medical Associations, and the American Cancer Society.

Prospective patients should begin by consulting their regular physician about medical marijuana. Many general practitioners are willing to write recommendations upon being informed that their patients find it relieves their symptoms. Others can be persuaded after being shown scientific evidence that marijuana is effective for the particular disease, such as the studies referred to in this book. Still other physicians will refuse entirely.

In this case, patients should exercise their legal right to request a copy of their medical records, which will at least document that they have been under medical treatment for a serious disease. They can then present their records to another doctor more knowledgeable about cannabis medicine. Specialists in cannabis medicine are now practicing in most states with medical marijuana laws. Referrals can generally be found on the Internet or from patient's groups in your state. Most cannabis specialists will require documentation showing prior treatment for the patient's complaint. If the disease is one that can be treated with cannabis and is covered by state law, most specialists will provide a recommendation following an appropriate examination.

States typically require that recommendations come from a physician who is licensed to practice in that state. An exception is Vermont, which allows recommendations by doctors from its three neighboring states. Occasionally, sympathetic courts in medical marijuana states will dismiss charges for patients with out-of-state recommendations. Montana is the only state with a law specifically recognizing medical marijuana ID or registry cards issued by other states.

Conditions Allowed

Most states have a restricted list of conditions for which medical marijuana may be legally used. The major exception is California, which allows marijuana to be recommended for "any illness for which marijuana provides relief." This is actually the current standard for FDA-approved drugs, all of which may be prescribed legally for any condition, regardless of whether it is listed on the label. However, because of marijuana's unique, controversial status under federal law, lawmakers have tried to restrict its use even though it is actually safer than most prescription drugs.

Typically, most states permit medical use of marijuana for the following categories of use:

1. Nausea (e.g. from chemotherapy)
2. Appetite loss or severe weight loss (e.g. from cancer or HIV)
3. Muscle spasms or seizures (e.g. from MS or epilepsy)
4. Chronic pain (the broadest category)
5. Glaucoma

Some states allow patients to petition for the inclusion of other conditions as well. A few specify that diseases be "severe" or "debilitating" or unresponsive to other treatments.

The standard indications cover most, but not all, uses of medical marijuana. Notably absent from the standard list are psychiatric and mood disorders like PTSD and bipolar disorder. Psychiatric recommendations constitute some 20% of the patient population in California, the only state where they are permitted.

Registration

Most states require patients to register with the state in order to enjoy protection of the law (exceptions are California, Washington, and Maine). In theory, registered patients are supposed to be protected from arrest if they follow the law. Certain states provide an affirmative defense for non-registered patients who happen to be arrested but can demonstrate their medical need in court. In this case, patients can defend themselves from criminal charges by bringing in a physician to testify that they had recommended medical marijuana. In order to enjoy protection of the law, patients need to have their doctor's recommendation before they are arrested.

Some patients are nervous about registering with the state due to fear that the information could be used to prosecute or harass them by the federal government. Fortunately, these fears have not been born out in practice. Not a single one of the thousands of patients who have registered in state medical marijuana programs has so far had their records turned over to federal authorities. Federal authorities have stated that they have no interest in pursuing individual patients.

In one instance, the U.S. attorney's office in Eastern Washington State tried to subpoena patient records from Oregon in order to pursue an investigation of a local cannabis clinic. U.S. District Court Justice Robert Whaley denied the request, ruling that patients' privacy concerns overrode the grand jury's need for information. The Washington case was not aimed at investigating patients, but rather a clinic. Had the government tried to prosecute actual patients, it would doubtless have faced even stronger legal and political resistance in light of the strong popular support for medical marijuana. Qualified patients should therefore have no fear about registering where possible in state programs to protect themselves from arrest by state authorities.

In some states without medical marijuana laws, seriously ill patients who have been arrested for personal possession or cultivation may be able to defend themselves in court by invoking an old common law doctrine known as the necessity defense. The necessity defense is applicable only in very narrow circumstances, where the defendant can prove that it was necessary to break the law in order to protect his or her life or health from greater imminent harm. The necessity defense is available only to the most gravely ill patients who have exhausted all other courses of medical treatment. Not all states allow for a necessity defense. Maryland, which does not otherwise allow medical marijuana or a necessity defense, has a law specifically allowing marijuana patients to invoke a necessity defense, in which case they are subject to no more than a $100 fine.

It has not been decided whether medical necessity is an allowable defense in federal court. In its Oakland Cannabis Buyers' Cooperative decision (2001), the US Supreme Court ruled that necessity was not a valid defense for third parties seeking to manufacture or distribute marijuana for others who had medical need for it. However, it left open the question of whether it might be allowable for individual patients charged with personal possession or cultivation. Since no necessity patients have ever been arrested for personal possession or cultivation by the federal government, the issue remains undecided.

Quantity Limits

Most states have established rather stingy limits on the quantity of marijuana patients can legally possess or cultivate. In some states, patients who have been arrested with larger amounts may still argue innocence in court by invoking an "affirmative defense," under which they must show that the higher quantities were medically justified for their own personal use. In other states, the limits are rigorously enforced.

Most states permit patients to possess no more than a few ounces.

This is typically less than the average patient's yearly needs. On average, most patients use a joint or so per day, or about one half to one pound of good quality sinsemilla per year. Many severely ill patients consume two or three pounds of sinsemilla or more. Patients who consume marijuana orally may use significantly higher quantities of lower-grade leaf. The patients in the government's compassionate use program receive over six pounds of marijuana per year from NIDA; the higher quantity reflects the fact that NIDA's marijuana consists of low potency leaf.

It is typically impossible for most patients to stay within the legal possession guidelines if they want to grow a whole year's supply from a single, outdoor crop. The alternative is to continually replenish their supply a few ounces at a time every couple of months, either by maintaining an indoor garden with rotating crops or by purchasing from underground suppliers.

The stingy cultivation limits allowed by most states pose a difficult hurdle to patients who wish to comply with the law. Most states allow no more than a half dozen plants. While six large plants may be sufficient in a good outdoor grow, only under carefully controlled conditions is it possible for a half dozen indoor plants to fulfill a patient's needs. The patient must maintain a rotating crop, with the maximum allowed number constantly growing, each crop with the proper total yield of a few ounces, and a backup supply of immature plants to take their place. All of this requires considerable skill, experience, and luck, along with the requisite supplies and growing space.

In short, current state laws do not provide a realistic or convenient framework for most patients to meet their medical needs. In practice, patients are often forced to cheat on the limits or else rely on outside suppliers.

Patient Cooperatives

An appealing alternative for patients who wish to comply with the law is to join or organize a cultivation co-op. (The right for patients to collectively cultivate together is generally implicit in state medical marijuana laws.) If several patients join together on a collective garden, sharing expenses, labor, and a common grow-space, it is easier to provide a consistent supply within the constraints of the law. The size of the garden can be scaled to the number of patients. Economies of scale make it easier for ten patients to grow thirty plants together than for each to grow three plants separately. The major problem in forming a co-op is organizational. Patients must somehow find other nearby patients to work with. Fortunately, in these days of the Internet it has become easier to do so. Interested patients can now search the web for cooperatives in their area.

Another problem with co-ops is that their size tends to attract interest from law enforcement. The larger the garden, the more likely it will be discovered, and the more likely that police will try to charge the proprietors with illegal cultivation or sale. Many of the more difficult medical marijuana cases tend to involve co-ops. When gardens begin running into the hundreds of plants, local authorities are also more likely to call in the DEA, using federal law to strip the defendants of any medical marijuana defense under state law. As of this writing, over 100 medical marijuana providers have faced federal charges, almost all of them in California, and it appears certain that more will do so before federal law is changed.

Ultimately, the most convenient solution for most patients would be to simply buy their marijuana from a store like any other medicine.

Medical Cannabis Dispensaries

This solution is currently available only in California, Canada, Colorado and a few other places that tolerate so-called medical cannabis dispensaries (*aka* compassion clubs or buyers clubs). Dispensaries are essentially stores where marijuana is sold to patients who have a doctor's recommendation. Most dispensaries will sell only to patients who are legal under state law, excluding those from out-of-state. Ironically, however, dispensaries themselves are not strictly legal under state or national law, even where they are tolerated by local authorities.

Dennis Peron, the organizer of California's Compassionate Use-Initiative, established the first public medical cannabis club in San Francisco in 1993, and pioneered the model for cannabis buyers clubs. The San Francisco Buyers' Club was loosely modeled on an Amsterdam coffee shop, with lounges, tables and chairs where members could socialize and smoke. Entry was restricted to members, who had to have a doctor's note showing their need for medical marijuana. Cannabis was sold at a "bud bar" with a menu of varieties, most commonly sold in eighths of an ounce (enough for 3 to 6 joints). Soft drinks and other refreshments were also available, as well as cannabis edibles. The club provided a variety of activities and social services—patient support groups, massage, a doctor's research group, meeting spaces, and recreational activities. It also became Peron's political headquarters for California's medical marijuana initiative, Prop. 215. Originally located in a modest upstairs space, the club relocated to a five-story building in downtown San Francisco in order to accommodate the growing number of patrons. At its height, the club served over 12,000 members, with visitors and media flocking from around the world to see medical marijuana dispensed in a friendly, accommodating, safe environment.

All of this occurred without any official legal sanction. The club opened up before California's medical marijuana law was passed, following the approval of a legally non-binding marijuana resolution by the city's voters, Proposition P (1991). Even after Prop. 215 passed, California law did not specifically permit distribution or sales of marijuana, only personal use and cultivation. Still, San Francisco city officials were highly supportive, and local police refused to bust Peron's club.

This tolerance did not extend to state officials, however, in particular Attorney General Dan Lungren, an archconservative opponent of California's medical marijuana law. On Lungren's orders, state narcotics agents raided Peron's club and eventually forced its closure. By this time, however, other dispensaries had begun to sprout up. Within a year after passage of Prop. 215, a dozen different dispensaries were in operation.

Alarmed by the spread of the dispensaries, federal officials swung into action. In 1998, the Department of Justice filed a lawsuit to close six of the most prominent dispensaries, led by Oakland's Cannabis Buyers' Cooperative. In court, advocates for the dispensaries argued that federal laws were inapplicable on the grounds that the dispensaries were not engaged in interstate commerce, that states had a right to legislate their own laws, and that marijuana was medically necessary to relieve pain and suffering for many patients. The district court rejected these arguments and issued an injunction to close the six dispensaries, including the OCBC. Although the ruling was partially reversed by the Ninth Circuit Court of Appeals, it was ultimately re-affirmed by the U.S. Supreme Court in 2001 (*U.S. v. Oakland Cannabis Buyers' Cooperative*).

Nonetheless, despite the closure of both the OCBC and Peron's club, medical marijuana dispensaries continued to flourish in California. Following the Supreme Court's ruling, there were more dispensaries than ever in the state. The federal government took another swipe at the dispensaries, raiding the only major one in Southern California, the LA Cannabis Resource Center, just weeks after 9/11. It went on to raid the state's leading cultivation cooperative, the Wo/Men's Alliance for Medical Marijuana, which served over 200 seriously ill patients in Santa Cruz. Still, the clubs proliferated. Tolerance for the dispensaries was aided by the election of a new attorney general in California, Bill Lockyer, who was openly sympathetic to medical marijuana. Despite the lack of clear legal sanction in state law, the official policy of the attorney general was to let local counties and cities permit medical cannabis dispensaries if they want to. Subsequently, some localities, including Oakland, San Francisco, and Los Angeles County, enacted ordinances officially regulating dispensaries despite their illegality under federal law. Other localities acted to ban them entirely.

The number of dispensaries began soaring after 2004, when hundreds of clubs began sprouting up in Los Angeles and Southern California. The DEA mounted a counteroffensive in 2007, raiding dozens of LA-area dispensaries and sending letters to their landlords warning that their premises could be subject to federal forfeiture. If history is any guide, there will likely be a retrenchment, followed by a resurgence, in dispensaries. As of this writing, there are over 250 dispensaries and co-ops in California, plus countless more home delivery services.

From time to time, federal agents continue to harass and occasionally arrest medical cannabis providers. In most cases, the targets are dispensaries that have become conspicuously big and profitable or which have antagonized local officials. Fortunately, in no case have the feds pursued the dispensaries' members or other legitimate patients.

For whatever reason, there remains a conspicuous lack of cannabis dispensaries in other states. However, there are a growing number of patients' support groups and co-ops that help patients cultivate or obtain medicine for themselves, in states including Oregon, Washington, Colorado, Hawaii, Montana and Rhode Island. In Canada, where medical use of marijuana is protected by a decision of the country's highest court, "compassion clubs" are operating publicly in a number of cities. At this point, it appears unlikely that the U.S. Justice Department will be able to put a halt to the spread of cannabis co-ops and dispensaries.

Shopping for Cannabis Dispensaries

Most cannabis dispensaries are now listed on the Internet at such websites as *www.canorml.org*. Many have websites of their own, and some even advertise in local newspapers.

Cannabis dispensaries come in many different varieties and flavors. Few operate on the grand scale of Peron's original dispensary or provide the same variety of services. Many operate as simple take-out stores, where patients come in, present their IDs, buy their medicine, and leave with no other services offered. Relatively few allow on-site consumption. Though local law frequently disallows smoking, some dispensaries offer vaporizers for use instead. Virtually all restrict their clientele to in-state residents who are legal under state law. Most require first-time patients to bring in their physician's recommendation to document their legality, though a few honor state or other patient ID cards. Most limit sales to no more than an ounce at a time so as to discourage illegal re-distribution.

Some offer cannabis extracts, tonics, oils, and hashish where permitted by local authorities. A dazzling array of edibles are

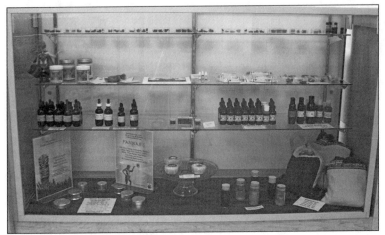

A medical cannabis dispensary counter in California.

available through the dispensaries, including cannabis-tainted cookies, brownies and cakes, candies, butter and cooking oil, ice cream, soda, even peanut butter and jelly. As always, it is difficult to judge the potency of edibles. Fortunately, commercial producers have arisen who manufacture edibles of consistent, predictable potency and who even have brand labels. Unfortunately, the industry has attracted adverse attention from the DEA, who have busted a couple of the largest producers.

Also unfortunately, there is absolutely no guarantee about the quality or purity of cannabis sold in the dispensaries. Federal laws have kept growers entirely underground, where it is impossible to monitor their use of pesticides, plant potency and cannabinoid content, plant strain, or adherence to organic standards. No dispensary can divulge the source of its marijuana, unless, as is sometimes the case, the dispensary's members grow it themselves. Customers must therefore rely on the dispensary's reputation or word of mouth.

Clones are one of the most valuable products that dispensaries can offer for patients to start their own gardens. Clones are a difficult product to carry, since they take up space and must be carefully maintained with light and water. Furthermore, the pos-

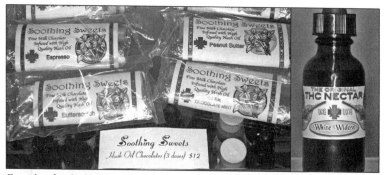

Examples of medical edibles and cannabis tinctures available at medical cannabis dispensaries.

session of 100 clones or more automatically exposes the owner to a federal mandatory minimum sentence of 5 years. It is legally safer to carry bulk marijuana, for which mandatory minimums don't kick in until one reaches the quantity of 100 kilos. Nevertheless, a number of dispensaries do offer clones at surprisingly affordable prices as low as $10 per clone, costing no more than a single joint.

Unfortunately, very few dispensaries offer seeds. Domestic supplies of seeds are scarce because most growers are wedded to growing seedless sinsemilla. The biggest suppliers of seeds are foreign companies from Canada and Europe. While their products can be ordered illegally on the Internet for anonymous mail shipment to the U.S., there are obvious legal risks in receiving them. The DEA is constantly on the lookout for foreign seed exporters, and has been known to intercept and seize their customer lists.

Patients and law enforcement officials alike often grumble about the high price of cannabis from the dispensaries. Prices typically run around $40 to $70 per eighth of an ounce – not very different from the illegal street price. The price of cannabis in the dispensaries reflects a host of costs involved in running the store – rent, wages, insurance, security, bookkeeping, even taxes (in California, medical marijuana is subject to sales taxes) – not to mention the increased costs imposed by federal prohibition. On the other hand, the dispensaries also deliver increased value to the customer – wider choice of products, a safer and more pleasant environment, and a reliable and accountable source to whom customers can complain in case the product is bad. It pays to shop around: prices vary widely among competing dispensaries. In the end, the market will out. Dispensaries that charge too much are eventually forced to close.

If you don't like the market price, your best option is to grow for yourself. In most states with medical marijuana laws, this is the only completely legal option. The problem, of course, is that it's easy to run afoul of the law, and even if you are operating entirely legally, you still risk arrest from malevolent cops. Even though cannabis dispensaries are illegal, there's no law against buying marijuana – only selling, growing, and possessing it. So weigh your options carefully and be aware of the risks.

Medical Marijuana State Laws

State	Conditions Allowed	Quantity Limit	Registration	Legislation Passed	# of Patients
Alaska	cachexia; cancer; chronic pain; epilepsy and other disorders characterized by seizures; glaucoma; HIV or AIDS; multiple sclerosis and other disorders characterized by muscle spasticity; and nausea. Other conditions are subject to approval by the Alaska Department of Health and Social Services	1 ounce; 6 plants (max 3 mature)	Yes	Mar. 1999	200 patients
California	any disease	8 ounces 6 mature or 12 immature plants (more by local option in some counties or by MD's exemption)	Voluntary IDs issued by county health depts	Nov. 1996	est. 250,000-350,000 patients
Colorado	cachexia; cancer; chronic pain; chronic nervous system disorders; epilepsy and other disorders characterized by seizures; glaucoma; HIV or AIDS; multiple sclerosis and other disorders characterized by muscle spasticity; and nausea. (Others may be approved by Board of Health)	2 ounces 6 plants*	Yes (*affirmative defense for those without IDs)	2001	3300 patients
Hawaii	cachexia; cancer; chronic pain; Crohn's disease; epilepsy and other disorders characterized by seizures; glaucoma; HIV or AIDS; multiple sclerosis and other disorders characterized by muscle spasticity; and nausea. (Others may be approved by Dept of Health)	1 ounce 7 plants, max. 3 mature	Mandatory IDs	Dec. 2000	4200 patients
Maine	epilepsy and other disorders characterized by seizures; glaucoma; multiple sclerosis and other disorders characterized by muscle spasticity; and nausea or vomiting as a result of AIDS or cancer chemotherapy	2.5 ounces 6 plants (max 3 mature)* Larger amounts treatable as simple possession	None	Dec. 1999	
Montana	cachexia or wasting syndrome; severe or chronic pain; severe nausea; seizures, including but not limited to seizures caused by epilepsy; or severe or persistent muscle spasms, including but not limited to spasms caused by multiple sclerosis or Crohn's disease.	6 plants	Yes Other state IDs recognized. 1 Caregiver per patient.	Nov. 2004	120 cards
Nevada	AIDS; cancer; glaucoma; and any medical condition or treatment to a medical condition that produces cachexia, persistent muscle spasms or seizures, severe nausea or pain. Others by approval of Dept of Human Resources.	1 ounce 7 plants (max 3 mature)*	Yes Required	2007	900 cards
New Mexico	"Debilitating" conditions: Cancer, glaucoma, MS, spinal injury, epilepsy, HIV, hospice patients. Others by approval of Dept of Health	Possession amounts to be determined; Cultivation by licensed producer – regulations under development	Yes *Affirmative defense for those without IDs	Oct. 2001	

Oregon	cachexia; cancer; chronic pain; epilepsy and other disorders characterized by seizures; glaucoma; HIV or AIDS; multiple sclerosis and other disorders characterized by muscle spasticity; and nausea. Others by approval of Dept of Human Resources	24 ounces 6 mature plants (18 immature seedlings) ABSOLUTE MAX	Yes Affirmative defense available without IDs	Nov. 1998	16,600 patients 8000 caregivers
Rhode Island	cachexia; cancer; glaucoma; Hepatitis C; severe, debilitating, chronic pain; severe nausea; seizures, including but not limited to, those characteristic of epilepsy; or severe and persistent muscle spasms, including but not limited to, those characteristic of multiple sclerosis or Crohn's Disease; or agitation of Alzheimer's Disease. Other conditions are subject to approval by the Rhode Island Department of Health.	2.5 ounces 12 plants (indoors only)	Yes Affirmative defense for others	Jan. 2006	192 patients
Vermont	Chronic or debilitating nausea, chronic pain, wasting, seizures, cancer, MS, HIV	2 ounces 2 mature + 7 immature plants	Yes	Jul 2004, amended Jun 2007	20 patients
Washington	cachexia; cancer; HIV or AIDS; epilepsy; glaucoma; intractable pain (unrelieved by standard treatment); and multiple sclerosis. Others of approval by state Board of Health inc. Crohn's Disease, Hep C, + any disease causing Nausea, seizures, appetite loss, muscle spasms unrelieved by standard treatment.	60-day supply	None Caregivers for 1 patient only.	Nov. 1998	

Appendix

Table 1: International Classification of Diseases 9–CM 1996 Chronic Conditions Treated With Cannabis Encountered Between 1990-2005
©2005 Tod H. Mikuriya, M.D.

Condition	Code	Condition	Code
AIDS Related Illness	042	Arthropathy, gout	274.0
Shingles (Herpes Zoster)	053.9	Mucopolysaccharoidosis	277
Genital Herpes	054.10	Porphyria	277.1
Herpetic infection of penis	054.13	Amyloidosis	277.3
Post W.E. Encephalitis	062.1	Obesity, exogenous	278.00
Chemotherapy Convalescence	V66.2	Obesity, morbid	278.01
Viral B Hepatitis, chronic	070.52	Autoimmune disease	279.4
Viral C Hepatitis, chronic	070.54	Thallasemia	282.4
Other arthropod borne dis.	088.	Hemophilia A	286.0
Lyme Disease	088.81	Henoch-Schoelein Purpura	287.0
Reiters Syndrome	099.3	Senile Dementia+	290.0
Behcet's Syndrome++	138.0	Delerium Tremens+	291.0
Osteoblastoma Ischium	170.6	Schizophrenia(s)	295.x
Malignant Melanoma	172.x	Schizoaffective Disorder	295.7
Other Skin Cancer	173	Mania	296.0
Breast Cancer	174.x	Major Depression, Sgl Epi	296.2
Prostate Cancer	185	Major Depression, Recurr	296.3
Prostate Cancer	186	Bipolar Disorder	296.6
Testicular Cancer	186.9	Autism/Aspergers	299.0
Adrenal Cortical Cancer	194.0	Anxiety Disorder+	300.00
Brain malignant tumor	191	Panic Disorder+	300.01
Glioblastoma Multiforme	191.9	Agoraphobia	300.22
Sarcoma: Head-neck	195.0	Obsessive Compulsive Dis.	300.3
Cancer, site unspecified	199	Dysthymic Disorder	300.4
Lympho- & reticulosacroma	200	Neurasthenia	300.5
Hodgkins disease	201.9	Impotence, Psychogenic	302.72
Myeloid leukemia	205	Alcoholism+	303.0
Uterine cancer	236.0	Opiate Dependence+	304.0
Lymphoma	238.7	Sedative Dependence+	304.1
Graves Disease**	242.0	Cocaine Dependence+	304.2
Acquired hypothyroidism	244	Amphetamine Depend.	304.4
Thyroiditis	245	Alcohol Abuse+	305.0
Diabetes Adult Onset	250.0	Tobacco Dependence	305.1
Diabetes Type I, Unctld ++	250.01	Psychogenic Hyperhidrosis	306.3
Diabetes Type I Ctrld ++	250.03	Psychogenic Pylorospasm**	306.4
Diabetes Insulin Depend.	250.1	Psychogenic Dysuria	306.53
Diabetes Adult Onset Unctrl	250.2	Bruxism	306.8
Diabetic Renal Disease	250.4	Stuttering*	307.0
Diabetic Ophthalmic Dis.	250.5	Anorexia Nervosa	307.1
Diabetic Neuropathy	250.6	Tic disorder unspec.	307.20
Diabetic PeripheralVasc. Dis.	250.7	Tourette's Syndrome	307.23
Hypoglycemia(s)	251	Persistent Insomnia	307.42
Lipomatosis	272.8	Nightmares	307.47

Bulemia	307.51	Optic neuritis	377.30
Tension Headache	307.81	Strabismus & other binoc. eye dis.	378
Psychogenic Pain	307.89	Nystagmus, Congenital	379.5
Post Traumatic Stress Dis.	309.81	Meniere's Disease	386.00
Mental Disorder,.head injury	310.1	Tinnitus	388.30
Post Concussion Syndrome	310.2	Hypertension+	401.1l
Nonpsychotic Org Brain Dis.	310.8	Ischemic Heart Disease	411.X
Brain Trauma	310.9	Angina pectoris	413
Intermittent Explosive Dis.	312.34	Arteriosclerotic Heart Dis.	414.X
Trichotillomania	312.39	Cardiac conduction disord.	426.X
ADD w/o hyperactivity	314.00	Paroxysmal Atrial Tach**	427.0
ADD w hyperactivity	314.01	Congestive Heart Failure	428.0
ADD other	314.8	Post Cardiotomy Syndrom	429.4
Psychogenic PAT	316.0	Raynaud's Disease	443.0
Parkinsons Disease	332.0	Thromboangiitis Obliterans	443.1
Huntingtons Disease+	333.4	Polyarteritis Nodosa	446.0
Restless legs syndrome	333.99	Acute Sinusitis	461.9
Friedreich's Ataxia	334.0	Chronic Sinusitis	473.9
Cerebellar Ataxia	334.4	Chronic Obst. Pulmon. Dis.	491.90
Spinal muscular atrophy	335.11	Emphysema	492.8
Amytrophic Lateral Scler	335.2	Asthma, unspecified	493.9
Other spinal cord disease	336	Pneumothorax, Spontaneo	512.8
Syringomyelia	336.0	Pulmonary Fibrosis	516.3
Reflex Sympath. Dystrophy	337.2	Cystic Fibrosis	518.89
Multiple Sclerosis	340.0	Dentofacial anomaly pain	524.
Other CNS demyelinating	341.	T.M.J Sydrome	524.60
Hemiparesis/hemiplegia	342	Gastro-Esophageal Rflx Dis.	530.81
Cerebral Palsy+	343.9	Acute Gastritis	535.0
Quadriplegia(s)	344.0x	Gastritis+	535.5
Paraplegia(s)	344.1x	Peptic Ulcer/Dyspepsia	536.8
Paralysis, unspecified	344.9	Colitis, Ulcerative	536.9
Epilepsy(ies)+	345.x	Pylorospasm Reflux	537.81
Grand Mal Seizures**	345.1	Regional Enteri & Crohns	555.9
Limbic Rage Syndrome**	345.4	Colitis+	558.9
Jacksonian Epilepsy**	345.5	Colon diverticulitis	562.1
Migraine(s)+	346.x	Constipation	564.0
Migraine, Classical+	346.0	Irritable Bowel Synd.	564.1
Cluster Headaches	346.2	Dumping Synd.. Post Surg	564.2
Compression of Brain	348.4	Peritoneal pain	568
Tic Douloureux+	350.1	Hepatitis-non-viral	571.4
Bell's palsy	351.0	Pancreatitis	577.1
Thoracic Outlet Synd.	353.0	Celiac disease	579.0
Phantom Limb Synd.++	353.6	Nephritis/nephropathy	583.81
Carpal Tunnel Syndrome	354.0	Ureter spasm calculus	592
Mononeuritis lower limb	355	Urethritis/Cystitis	595.3
Charcot-Marie-Tooth Synd.	356.1	Prostatitis	600.0
Neuropathy+	357	Epididymitis**	604.x
Muscular dystrophies	359	Pelvic pain	607.9
Coat's Syndrome++	362.12	Testicular torsion	608.2
Macular Degeneration**	362.5	Pelvic Inflammatory Dis.	614
Glaucoma	365.23	Endometriosis**	617.9
Dyslexic Amblyopia**	368.0	Premenstrual Syndrome+	625.3
Color Blindness*	368.55	Pain, Vaginal/Pelvic	625.9
Conjuctivitis	372.9	Menopausal syndrome	627.2
Drusen of Optic Nerve	377.21	Sturge-Weber Disease	759.6

Eczema	692.9	Marfan syndrome	759.82
Pemphigus	694.4	Sturge-Weber Eye Syn**	759.6
Epidermolysis Bullosa	694.9	Nater's Syndrome++	759.89
Erythma Multiforma	695.1	Insomnia+	780.52
Rosacea	695.3	Sleep Apnea Unspecified	780.57
Psoriatic Arthritis	696.0	Chronic Fatigue Synd	780.7
Psoriasis	696.1	Tremor/Invol Movements	781.0
Pruritis, pruritic+	698.9	Myofacial Pain Syndrme**	782.0
Neurodermatitis	698.3	Anorexia+	783.0
Atrophy Blanche	701.3	Bulemia	783.6
Alopecia	704.x	Hyperventilation	786.01
Lupus	710.0	Cough+	786.2
Scleroderma	710.1	Hiccough+	786.8
Sjogren's Disease++	710.2	Vomiting	787.01
Dermatomyositis	710.3	Nausea+	787.02
Eosinophilia-Myalgia Syn.	710.5	Diarrhea	787.91
Arthritis, Rheumatoid+	714.0	Pain, Ureter	788.0
Felty's Syndrome	714.1	Cachexia	799.4
Arthritis, Degenerative	715.0	Vertebral disloc unspec .	839.4
Arthritis, post traumatic+	716.1	Whiplash	847.0
Arthropathy, Degenerat+	716.9	Back Sprain	847.9
Patellar chondromalacia	717.7	Shoulder Injury Unspec	959.2
Ankylosis	718.5	Fore Arm/Elbow/Wrist	959.3
Multiple joints pain	719.49	Hand except finger	959.4
Intervertebral Disk Disease	722.x	Finger injury	959.5
L-S disk dis sciatic N irrit	722.1	Hip injury	959.6
IVDD Cerv w Myelopathy	722.71	Knee, ankle & foot injury	959.7
Cervical Disk Disease	722.91	Radiation Therapy	990
Cervicobrachial Syndrome	723.3	Motion Sickness	994.6
Lumbosacral Back Diseas	724.x	Anaphylactic or Reaction	995.0
Spinal Stenosis	724.02	Renal Transplant ++	996.81
Lower Back Pain	724.5		
Peripheral enthesopathies	726	+ Represents citations from pre-1937
Tenosynovitis	727.x	medical literature
Dupuytens Contracture	728.6	++ Jeffrey Hergenrather, M.D.
Muscle Spasm	728.85	* Eugene Schoenfeld, M.D.
Fibromyagia/Fibrositis	729.1	** Dale Gieringer, Ph.D. CANORML
Weber-Christian Dis.++	729.30	Hotline
Legg Calve Perthe Dis.++	732.1		
Osgood-Schlatter	732.4		
Osteoporosis	733.0		
Tietze's Syndrome	733.6		
Melorheostosis	733.99		
Spondylolisthesis**	738.4		
Cerebral Aneurism	747.81		
Polycystic Kidney	753.1x		
Scoliosis	754.2		
Club foot	754.70		
Spina Bifida Occulta	756.17		
Osteogenesis imperfecta	756.51		
Ehlers Danlos Syndrome	756.83		
Nail patella syndrome	756.89		
Peutz-Jehgers Syndrome**	756.9		
Mastocytosis	757.33		
Darier's Disease	757.39		

Bibliography

Lester Grinspoon & James B. Bakalar, *Marihuana, the Forbidden Medicine.* Yale U Press, 1997.

Franjo Grotenhermen & Ethan Russo, ed. *Cannabis and Cannabinoids: Pharmacology, Toxicology, and Therapeutic Potential.*Haworth Press, NY 2002.

Geoffrey Guy, Brian Whittle and Philip Robson, ed, *The Medicinal Uses of Cannabis and Cannabinoids.* Pharmaceutical Press, London 2004.

Paul Armentano, *"Emerging Clinical Applications for Cannabis and Cannabinoids: A Review of the Recent Scientific Literature 2000-2006,"* NORML/NORML Foundation (2007).

Janet Joy, Stanley Watson and John Benson, Jr, ed, *Marijuana and Medicine: Assessing the Science Base,* Institute of Medicine, National Academy Press, Washington DC 1999 (report commissioned by Office of National Drug Control Policy).

Tod Mikuriya, ed., *Marijuana Medical Papers 1839-1972* Medi-Comp Press, Oakland, CA 1973 (anthology of classic papers on medical cannabis).

O'Shaughnessy's: *The Journal of Cannabis in Clinical Practice.* http://www.ccrmg.org/journal.html

Sidney Cohen and Richard Stillman, ed., *The Therapeutic Potential of Marihuana.* Plenum Publishing, NY 1976.

Ethan Russo, ed. *Cannabis Therapeutics in HIV/AIDS (Journal of Cannabis Therapeutics Vol 1 #3/4).* Haworth Books, 2001.

Ethan Russo, Melanie Dreher, Mary Lynn Mathre, ed. *Women and Cannabis: Medicine, Science and Sociology.* (Journal of Cannabis Therapeutics Vol 2 #3/4), Haworth Books, 2002.

Mary Lynn Mathre, ed. *Cannabis in Medical Practice: A Legal, Historical and Pharmacological Overview of the Therapeutic Use of Mari-*

juana. McFarland Publications, Jefferson, N. Carolina 1997.

R.C. Randall, ed. *Marijuana, Medicine & The Law.* Galen Press, Washington, DC.

Vol 1: *Direct Testimony of Witnesses in hearings before DEA* (1988).

Vol 2: *Legal Briefs, Oral Arguments and Decision of the DEA Administrative Law Judge* (1989).

Vol 3: *Cancer Treatment & Marijuana Therapy: Marijuana's Use in the Reduction of Nausea and Vomiting and for Appetite Stimulation in Cancer Patients, Testimony from Historic Federal Hearings on Marijuana's Medical Use* (1990).

Vol 4: *Muscle Spasm, Pain & Marijuana Therapy, Testimony from Federal and State Court Proceedings* (1991).

General Books on Marijuana

Ed Rosenthal, Steve Kubby, and S. Newhart, *Why Marijuana Should Be Legal.* Thunder's Mouth Press, NY 2003.

Leslie Iversen, *The Science of Marijuana.* Oxford Press, 2000.

Mitch Earleywine, *Understanding Marijuana: A New Look at the Scientific Evidence.* Oxford Press, 2002.

Lynn Zimmer and John Morgan, *Marijuana Myths, Marijuana Facts: A Review of the Scientific Evidence.* Lindesmith Center, NY, 1997.

Lester Grinspoon, *Marihuana Reconsidered.* Harvard U. Press 1971.

Ernest Abel, *Marihuana: The First Twelve Thousand Years.* Plenum Press, NY 1980.

Ricardo Cortes, *It's Just a Plant.* Magic Propaganda Mill, Jan 2005.

Cultivation and Processing

Ed Rosenthal, *The Big Book of Buds Volume 3.* Quick American, Oakland, CA 2007.

Ed Rosenthal, *The Best of Ask Ed.* Quick American, Oakland, CA 2003.

Ed Rosenthal and S. Newhart, *Ask Ed: Marijuana Gold—Trash to Stash.* Quick American, Oakland, CA 2002.

Ed Rosenthal, *Easy Marijuana Gardening.* Quick American, Oakland, CA 2000.

SeeMoreBuds, *Marijuana Buds For Less: Grow 8 oz. of Bud for Less Than $100.* Quick American, Oakland, CA 2007.

Soma, *Organic Marijuana Soma Style.* Quick American, Oakland, CA 2005.

DJ Short, *Cultivating Exceptional Cannabis.* Quick American, Oakland, CA 2003.

Tom Flowers, *Marijuana Herbal Cookbook.* Rosetta Books, Oakland CA 1995.

Robert Connell Clark, *Hashish!* Red Eye Press, Los Angeles, 1998.

Michael Starks, *Marijuana Chemistry: Genetics, Processing & Potency.* Ronin Publishing, Berkeley, 1990.

History of Medical Marijuana Politics

Alan Bock, *Waiting to Inhale: The Politics of Medical Marijuana.* Seven Locks Press, Santa Ana, CA 2000.

Larry Sloman, *Reefer Madness: A History of Marijuana.* St. Martin's, Griffin, NY 1998 (2nd edition).

Wendy Chapkis and Richard Webb, *Dying to Get High: Marijuana as Medicine,* NY Univ. Press, 2008.

Organizations and Websites

International Association for Cannabis Medicine. European-based research group offers members access to issues of Journal of Cannabis Therapeutics (2001-2004). Website provides comprehensive coverage of latest scientific research: *http://www.cannabis-med.org/english/home.htm*.

Americans for Safe Access. National member-based organization devoted to legislation, education, litigation, grassroots actions and advocacy for medical marijuana patients and providers: *http://safe-accessnow.org*

NORML (National Organization for Reform of Marijuana Laws). Public interest group devoted to marijuana law reform offers consumer info, legal guidance, plus timely and informative summaries of latest scientific research: *http://www.norml.org*

California NORML. Co-sponsor of Prop 215—website includes comprehensive listing of medical marijuana physicians and providers: *http://www.canorml.org*

California Cannabis Research Medical Group. Organization of practicing medical cannabis physicians; publishes informative newspaper, O'Shaughnessy's: The Journal of Cannabis in Clinical Practice: *http://www.ccrmg.org/journal.html*

Drug War Facts. A website that provides reliable information pertaining to public health and criminal justice issues: *http://www.drugwarfacts.org*

Drug Sense. Comprehensive index of online drug news clips: *http://www.drugsense.org*.

Schaffer Library of Drug Policy. Historical documents, books and periodicals about the war on drugs: *http://www.druglibrary.org/schaffer*

Green Aid. The medical marijuana legal defense and education fund: *http://www.green-aid.com*

Marijuana Policy Project. Leading national sponsor of ballot initiatives and lobbying campaigns to reform marijuana laws: *http://www.mpp.org*

Patients Out of Time. Science-based educational forum sponsors conferences on therapeutic cannabis: *http://www.medicalcannabis.com*

Medical Marijuana Pro-Con. Website provides balanced discussion of issues: *http://www.medicalmarijuanaprocon.org*

Research on marijuana's medical use advances constantly. Current developments along with legal and policy changes are posted at

www.norml.org

Index